Buffalo Production System for Milk, Meat (Buffen) and Employment

About the Author

Prof. Nityanand Pathak has vast experience of teaching and research on various aspects of buffalo production. He established buffalo nutrition laboratory as Indian Veterinary Research Institute, Izatnagar. In the capacity of Diplomat and Project Leader he Worked for two years (1982-84) at the Buffalo and Pasture Research Center at Song Be in Ben Cat Province near Ho Chi Minh City of S.R. Vietnam. The team established research laboratories and research work. Prof. Pathak in the capacity of Director, Central Institute for Research on Buffalo, Hissar assurred round the year adequate green foods production at the Institutes farm. He is author and coauthor of 20 books published by different houses. The vastness of experience can be judged by his more then 150 co-workers and co-authors in Bharat and other countries.

Buffalo Production System for Milk, Meat (Buffen) and Employment

Nityanand Pathak

Former Director,
Central Institute for Research on Buffalo (CIRB), Hisar,
Former Project Leader,
Buffalo Research Centre, Song Be, Ven Cat, S.R. Vietnam
Former Vice President
Indian Society for Buffalo Development (ISBD), Hissar

SSPH

SATISH SERIAL PUBLISHING HOUSE

403, Express Tower, Commercial Complex
Azadpur, Delhi-110033 (India)
Phone : 011-27672852, Fax : 91-11-27672046
e-mail : info@satishserial.com, hkjain1975@yahoo.com
Website : www.satishserial.com

Published by :

SATISH SERIAL PUBLISHING HOUSE

403, Express Tower, Commercial Complex, Azadpur, Delhi-110033 (INDIA)
Phone : 011-27672852 Fax : 91-11-27672046
E-mail : info@satishserial.com, hkjain1975@yahoo.com

ISBN 978-93-86200-47-1

Composed, Designed & Printed in India

Preface

Buffalo production is a vast subject of animal husbandry. This maultipurpose domestic beast plays very important role in the management of food and nutrition security. Draught power and organic droppings of buffaloes are used for the cultivation of basal staple foods and sugarcane. The females produce milk of high feeding value and contribution is more than half of the total milk production in Bharat. The nutritional contribution of buffaloes will further increase on the comparison of protein and energy (milk fat) production. International demand of buffalo milk is increasing for the production of 'Mozarella cheese'. Another highly nutritious proteinous food is buffen (buffalo meat). Its consumption is increasing due to more balanced essential amino acids content and low fat and cholesterol content in the flesh. The demand of buffeal (bufeen veal) is also increasing and it has high export market but at the present level of per capita milk production, Bharat can not afford buffalo production requiring about six kilogram(me) of whole buffalo milk for one kilogram(me) gain. However, weaned buffalo calves of 8-12 months of age can be fattened to 300-350 kg body weight before 2 years of age.

Large varieties of sweets are prepared from the buffalo milk. Important cultured foods are dahi, yoghurt and srikhand. People of Punjab, Haryana, Gujarat, Western Uttar Pradesh and rural Delhi consume large quantity of liquid whole milk.

Different cottage and large scale commercial houses are producing varicty of household goods, leather, leather goods and other fancy articles of horns and long hairs of tail switch. Fat of hoovcs yield precious neat oil. The buffaloes provide large number of employment for almost all classes of people without bar of education, gender, cast, creed and skill etc. The employment is available from buffalo production to buffalo products processing and marketing.

In the presentation of this book, it is not fair for me to forget the selfless role of my grand father late Sh. Ram Jhalak Pathak and younger brother late Sh. Ram Sakal Pathak, small farmers, great grand mother Late Rajkali Devi, bhua late Dilshwari and Phupha Ji late Ram Sakal Pandey. All encouraged and provided environment for acquiring education. Post graduate education is the outcome of the hardship and sacrifice of late Susheela (March 11, 1967 to March 4, 2004). I received solace from grand children Ananya, Anshuman, Anuvarata, Adiya, Amulya, Atharva and Anavartika and most of the time Ananya and Anuvrat cared for my comfort. Special thanks to Dr. S.K. Saha for keen interest in publication of this Book. Sh. Harish Chandra Singh and Sh. R.C. Malhotra were always ready for finalizing the text.

Nityanand Pathak

Contents

1

Introduction

Buffaloes

Domestic buffaloes had been one of the major sources of power for agricultural operations in the humid-hot Asian countries of tropical and sub-temperate zones. These buffaloes are also greater contributors of nutritious milk and meat not only in the Asian countries of Europe. Africa and Americas. In Australia, Asian buffaloes specially swamp type are reared exclusively for meat production as a feral beast on the tall growing grasses of wet region of north-west provinces. The wild drarf buffaloes, Anoa (*bubalus bubalis depresiomis*) and Tamraw (*Bubalus bubalis mindorensis*) are now endangered species due to indiscriminate hunting for meat and byproducts. Now, these two drarf (pygmy) species are protected animals. African or Savanah native buffaloes, the large black buffaloes (*Syncerus caffer*) and small size red or forest buffaloes (*Syncerus nanus*) with their many sub-species could not be domesticated. Before the restriction of hunting and conservation in National Parks, these buffaloes were important game beast of Africa. These were hundred mainly for the heavy long horns of valuable trophies. The other products of food values were flesh, glands and blood, and hide was used for leather making.

Domestic Buffaloes (*Bubalus bubalis*)

Domestic buffaloes are primarily the native of humid-hot Asian countries, which spread to adjoining regions of neighbouring countries. Nomadic group of medieval period were probably carried domestic buffaloes. This was due to docile nature, amicable behaviour and high adaption in different agro-climatic conditions bestowed with edible herbage and water. Two types of domestic water buffaloes are (1) Indian dairy or riverine buffaloes (*Bubalus bubalis bubalis*) evolved in several breeds for large quantity milk yield of high fat (6-12%) content; and (2). Asian swamp buffaloes (*Bubalus bubalis swampis*) of agricultural power. Earlier in almost all Asian countries domestic buffaloes were eliminated from the system only after caesation of reproduction or chronic sterility in the females and retirement from work due to senile inefficiency. In other countries riverine buffaloes were raised for milk and meat.

All breeds of Indian riverine buffaloes (*Bubalus bubalis bubalis*) except the Toda breed of Neel giri region are dairy animals yielding 1200 to 300 kg milk during the lactation period of 305 days (Ranjhan and Pathak, 1979). In india swamp buffaloes (*Bubalus bubalis swampis*) have been also evolved as a multipurpose animal for power, milk, meat and by products. Milk yield of swamp buffaloes of Assam and sister states yield 500 to 900 kg sparable milk for human consumption during lactation period of 200-300 days (Singh, 1978; Tamuli, 1978). The increasing acceptance of buffalo milk in the east and south-east Asian countries was an important factor for the operation of crossbreeding programme between Indian dairy breeds specially the Murrah and Nili-Ravi breeds, which were taken away from India and Pakistan in China, Phillipines, Socialist Republic of Vietnam, Thailand, Laos and many other countries for the establishment of pure herds and also crossbred herds primarily for the milk and meat production. The author along with his coworkers from India and Vietnam established a Murrah based Buffalo Production Institute in a remote area of southern part of Vietnam during 1982-84. The Institute is situated on a large farm at Song Be in the Ben Cat Province of S.R. Vietnam about 90 km away from the Ho Chi Minh City. Different crosses are produced in these countries for milk and meat production. Now in most of the countries restrictions on the slaughter of buffaloes have been relaxed and now a days males are also fattened for meat (buffen) and veal type meat (buffeal) production. This shift took place due to extensive use of mechanical and oil driven implements in agro-industrial operations like ploughing, harvesting, thrashing and transportation of agricultural product to markets, mills and go-downs etc.

Buffalo production systems

In the Bhartiya subcontinent different extensive and semi-extensive systems of buffalo production are practiced. Being docile and easily adaptable in different less comfortable management, the buffaloes are preferred daily animals. Buffalo milk is also in high demand.

Foods from buffaloes

Buffalo milk is a highly nutritious food of good quality, complete protein and energy, and satisfactory source of minerals and vitamins. The Asian buffaloes have been translocated to almost all the continents for milk and meat production, particularly in the humid-hot tropical and sub-temperate countries. Large number of people of the Indian sub-continent prefers to drink sweetened buffalo milk. It is a common practice to sell boiling buffalo (also at some places mixed or cow milk) milk on the sides of roads and streets of the towns of Bharat and Pakistan, and also in the tarai towns of Nepal and few towns of Bangladesh. Erthen numbers and mini pictures (*Kulhad or Bharkuka or chukka*) are preferred for the drinking of milk because new mud pots from hearth (awan) imparts characteristic flavor of roasted mud pot to milk. Majority of people in the twons drink 250 ml to 500 ml sweetened hot boiling milk with a small piece of thick milk skin (malai) placed on the top of fluid milk in the tumbler. Milk is taken by majority of the people after dinner. However, children are encouraged to take milk twice daily. The quantity normally ranges from half to one litre daily. However, a small group of young boys in some areas are trained for wrestling and kabbadi and they are trained to consume 2 to 5 litres fluid milk or partly fluid milk and partly rabri (partially dehydrated milk in pans placed on direct fire).

Dahi (curd) is an important preparation of cultured milk. Dahi is used in different forms and most common in churning for the separation of butter (*makhan*) which is consumed fresh with other floods or heat treated for the manufacture of ghee (samna). The fluid curd left after the separation of butter is called "*chhanchh*" or "matha" and used as cold beverage or roti is soaked at the time of eating for increasing palatability. *Chhanchh* is quite common among the farmers since time immemorial. It was also offered to young calves and sour matha is used for the treatment of diarrhea in humans and pre-ruminant calves, kids, lambs and floats etc. In the summer season cold matha is taken for protection from the heat stress of summer. It is also used for the preparation of sour Indian foods like *cudhi, dahi-bara,* curd sour rice etc. after recognition of the probiotic value of lactobacilli, the food value of curd and matha has increased many fold. Now curd, *matha* and spiced salted matha are being marketed as beverages in polypacks of different sizes.

Milk is used for the preparation of basic products like khoa, chhenna, cream, butter and paneer, which are used for the preparation of different varieties of area specific sweets.

Edible flesh is the another nutritious low fat and low cholesterol containing food from buffaloes. Earlier buffalo meat was considered as a low quality food of animal origin but its detailed chemical analysis revealed the superiority of protein component. The buffalo meat Is a richer source of essential amino acids in comparison to meat of many other species of farm animals. For sometime male buffaloes and sterile females became burden on the owners due to extensive use of machine power in agriculture. The recognition of nutritional superiority of the buffalo meat (buffen) and buffalo veal or Buveal increased the demand and value. Now male3 buffalo calf rearing is remunerative and it has come as a relief for the young male buffalo calves. The buffalo calves are now attracting the attention of owners and mostly not being started to die. Studies have also revealed production of high quality 'baby bufveal' below 3 months and 'bufveal' at 6 months of age. Production of buffeal in Indian may increase on increased production of milk or on the development of a good quality, palatable milk replacer of comparable feeding value of the whole milk.

Although different varieties of sweets and other edible products are prepared from the buffalo milk, and several products from the buffalo carcass, but most of the people nationally and internationally are not well exposed. In order to increase the awareness about the quality and food values of milk and meat products, this concise book has been architected in six chapters comprising of introduction, mammary glands and lactation, milk and milk products, meat and meat products, valuable by products of buffalo production and their commercial utilization and employment around buffalo.

By-products of buffaloes

Valuable by products obtained from the slaughter of buffaloes provide basic raw material for different industries. The hide is used for the production of good quality leather, which is utilized for the manufacture of leather goods for inland markets and export. Whole blood collected from the buffaloes is used by the pharmaceutical industries for the preparation of serum and serum proteins. Different endocrine glands are processed by the pharmaceutical industries for the manufacture of hormones and enzymes. Bile is used for the manufacture of bile salts.

Different offal not eaten by humans and residue of blood and glands left after the extraction of hormones, enzymes and other valuable biochemical are utilized by the compounded feed manufacturing industry for the preparation of animal protein supplements used in the compounded feeds of poultry, pigs, dogs, cats and fishes.

The heavy horns are utilized for the manufacture of fancy articles, toys, key rings, walking sticks, spoons for the chemical laboratories, combs, hair pins and a variety of decoration items. Hooves are processed for the manufacture of coat button and hair clips. The fatty extract of horns is used as lubricant. Oil extracted from the hoof join is a valuable lubricant for the sophisticated machineries because it remains liquid at very low temperature.

Buffalo farming from rearing to production of variety of edible and non-edible commercial products followed by the marketing provides employment of different categories. It provides employment for illiterate layman to highly qualified technical personnel.

Employments from buffaloes

Buffaloes provide opportunities for large number of skilled as well as unskilled people from rural to urban ares. Buffaloes provide different kinds of basic products like milk and meat and byproducts from the cottage and mechanized industries. This main areas of employment can be classified into the following categories.

1. **Buffalo farming:** It provides employment for grazing, feeding, grooming, milking, cleaning and disposal of dung etc.
2. **Dairy production:** Production of fermented, condensed, coagulated and dehydrated milk products.

3. **Meat production** includes slaughter, dressing, dissection, grading and disposal of products, by products and wastes.
4. **Leather industry:** It ranges from small scale cottage industry of rural artisan to large scale tanneries.
5. Leather goods manufacturing industries.
6. Biochemical and pharmaceutical industries.
7. Marketing of the products.

Employment in associated areas

For running the buffalo farm and industries handling buffalo products and by products, different equipments and appliances are required. These produced by small scale local artisans and advance industries. Some of the potential employment providing areas can be listed as follows:

1. Fodder production and supply.
2. Compounded feed production and supply.
3. Mineral mixture and feed additives production and supply.
4. Cottage industry for handling, restraining and decoration of buffaloes.
5. Cold chain equipment production, supply and maintenance.
6. Farm and daily equipments production and supply.
7. Agricultural equipments and appliances production and supply.
8. Vehicle of different kinds for transportation of various products and other material.
9. Fodder seed production and fertilizer manufacture.

Conclusion

On the basis of increasing areas of water buffalo farming it can be visualized that high adaptability, easier management, docile nature, high class nutritious food production and high traction power have tremendously increased the global acceptance. Now domestic water buffaloes, both riverine type dairy breeds (*Bubalus bubalis or bubalus bubalis bubalis*) of the Bhartiya subcontinent and draught type swamp buffalo (Bubalus earabanensis or Bubalus swampis or Bubalus bubalis swampis) are one of the most wanted species of domestic animals. All breeds of domestic buffaloes are the animals of wet land but they are successfully reared in the dry areas and also in many parts of the temperate zones provided there are adequate supply of water for drinking and bath or wallowing.

Growing increase in the consumption of mozrella cheese is increasing the demand of buffalo milk. Best mozella cheese of wide acceptability is prepared from the buffalo milk. The population of dairy breeds is increasing and spreading in many countries. The male calves earlier used for draught are now fattened young for buffeal (Buffalo veal) and buffen (similar to beef). The nutritional quality of buffeal and buffen is much superior in terms of essential amino acids, in comparison to meat of the most mammalian species.

Different kinds of by products particularly that obtained from the slaughtered buffaloes are valuable material for the leather and leather utilizing industries, pharmaceutical industries, biochemical industries and feed supplements manufacturing industries. No part of buffalo body is wastes. Dung, urine and other organic wastes of the buffalo farms are good sources of manure for improving the fertility of the agricultureal lands. In few words it can be concluded that buffaloes will grow for providing nutritious feeds and byproducts of industrial uses. It has enormous employment potential for all classes of people illiterate to highly educated, non-technical to technical, school going children to senior citizens without any gender bias.

References

Pathak, N.N. 2014. Buffaloes of the world and domestic water buffaloes. IBDC, Lucknow.

Pathak, N.N. 1996. Nutrition and feeding of male buffalo calves for the production of meat (Buffen) and working animals. Pub. No. 34, Indian Veterinary Research Institute, Izatnagar.

Ranjhan, S.K. and Pathak, N.N. 1989. A text book of Buffalo Production. 4th edn. Vikas Publishing House Pvt. Ltd. New Delhi.

Singh, D. 1978, M.V. Sc. Thesis, Assam Agril. University, Khanapara.

Tamuli, B.C., 1978. M.V.Sc. Thesis, Assam Agril, University, Khanapara.

❑❑❑

2

Buffalo Production Systems

Introduction

In the diet of predominant vegetarian population of Indian people the milk and milk products are the only source of good quality protein supply of animals origin. The milk has been recognized as vegetarian food since ancient times in India and even the strict vegetarians consume milk and milk products without any inhibition. Buffaloes have been evolvewd as a main dairy animal in India since the initiation of their domestication during epic period of Ramayan and Mahabharat (about 6000-5000 BC) which was probably completed during the Indus valley civilization period about (2200-1600 BC). Asian buffaloes are considered to be evolved from the Bubalus palaeindicus of the Plicene period. Indian domestic buffaloes are believed to be the descendent of wild arna buffalo (*Bubalus bubalis arnee*) present even today in the forests of north eastern states, forests of central India, western region and probably also in the sourthern region, but some conspicuous morphological differences appear to be the indication of the existence of atleast two (if not more) varieties of ancestors-one without chevron and ark colour with or without whiel marking like Murrah, Nili-Ravi, Kundi, Zaffarabadi and in my opinion also Mehsana. The wild ancestors of these breeds are no more found in any part of Indian sub-contient; the other with one to three chevrons are found in wild in river basins and other water source of the fores, probably domesticated breeds possessing one to three chevrons like Surti, Pandharpuri, Nagpuri, Toda, Bhadawari and at least one strain of Tarai and some breeds of Orissa are the descendents of present day wild arni (*Bubalus bubalis arnee*). All swamp buffalo buffaloes including those found in India except the valley type of Manipur display chevrons and also considered to be the descendent of arni but number of chromosomes of dairy type river buffaloes 92n=50) and that of swamp buffaloes (2n=48) indicate the existence of separate ancestor which is perhaps also extinct. The origin of Mehsana from interbreeding between Murrah and Surti was first time pronounced by Oliver (1938). The basis of this is perhaps not known even today. However, this claim has been endorsed several times (ICAR, 1941;

Mason, 1969; Cockrill, 1974; Ranjhan and Pathak, 1979; Acharya, 1991). The chevrons are even recessive traits the chances of its occasional appearance in a Mehsana herd is expected but it is not seen., Therefore, there is need of defining all breeds of modern buffaloes distributed throughout the country.

Distribution of Domesticated Buffaloes in Bharat (India)

Domesticated buffaloes primarily reared for milk production are distributed right from Kanyakumari in south to the Bugyals above Shri Kedarnath at the height over 4000 m in north, and Jammu and Kashmir in west to hilly states of north-eastern region. Local small size buffaloes are also found in Andaman and Nicobar islands. The domesticated buffaloes may be distributed into two broad groups of describing the production system.

Types of Domesticated Buffaloes

The two main types are diary type riverine buffaloes and multipurpose swamp buffaloes.

A. Riverine (dairy type) buffaloes

These are represented by several well defined and a few occasionally defined breeds and may be grouped into following subclasses:

1. **Murrah group of buffaloes:** These are mostly heavy breeds of black buffaloes evolved in the northern and western part of the country extending from Gujarat to Punjab. These breeds may possess white marking and occasionally there may be brown specimen but they do not possess chevron at any stage during post-natal life. There is probably no record of the prenatal status. Murrah, Nili-Ravi, Kindi, Jaffarabadi and Mehsana may be included in the Murrah group of buffaloes and all these breeds are famous for high milk production of rich better fat content not only in India but also to many other countries.

2. **Breeds of central belt of India:** Extending from Gujarat to Orissa and also some parts of northern states, most of the breeds are modeium sized, good milk yielders, widely adaptable to harsh agro climatic conditions, generally lighter in colour and in most of the breeds one to three chevrons are present well recognized

brees in this group are Surti, Pandharpuri, Napuri, Bhadawari, Tarai (atleast one strain) and relatively less known breeds of Orissa like sambalpuri, Peddakimedi, Parlimedi, Bheda, Kujan, Parikad, manda and Jerangi.

3. **Breeds of south Indian:** During visits to south India author has been the small scattered groups of similar buffaloes in all the states down the Nagpur but except the description of Toda and South Kanara probably no attempt has been made to describe the native buffaloes of the region whereas existence of large size buffaloes in the region has shown in Ramayan. Lately, a variety of dairy buffalo in Andhara Pradesh is being mentioned as Godawari breed and its evolution is being claimed from the inter se natural breeding between local and Murrah for many generations.
4. **Dairy buffaloes of north-east states:** Perhaps no attempt has been made to differentiate the buffaloes o north-east states extending from Sikkim and adjoining areas of West Bengal to bordering states of India i.e. Arunachal Pradesh, Mizoram, Manipur, Nagaland, Tripura and Meghalaya although all states are having one or more type of buffaloes and it is expected that some of them may be widely distributed in all the state. The native buffaloes of these stares are being classified as swamp buffaloes but large number of dairy buffaloes are also found. These buffaloes were introduced by Mughals and later on by the Britishers from the north Indian states of modern dairy buffaloes of these states are the complex mixture evolved from the inter breeding of river and swamp as well as occasional mating with wild males. Thus, it has become very difficult to describe the dairy buffaloes kept in the urban and peri-urban areas for milk production.
5. **Buffaloes of Andaman and Nicobar Islands:** There are small native buffaloes and record of their origin is perhaps not available. All attempts of inhabitating dairy buffaloes from main land has failed.

B. Swamp (draught type) buffaloes

These are domesticated and also some tamed type of buffaloes reared in different north-east Indian states. Existence of swamp buffaloes has been mentioned in some other states also, but basis of such statements has not been given. These are mainly kept for milk production followed by draught and meat production.

Scattered small herds or groups 1 to 10 animals are reared in the hilly region of Jammu and Kashmir, Himanchal Pradesh, Uttarakhand, Sikkim and also in hilly region of north-eastern states and so far no knowledge is available about their evolution and linkages with the other Indian buffaloes. These are also either domesticated or tamed buffaloes but almost all are lighter in size and narrower in shape with strong foot hold.

Purpose of Buffalo Rearing

About two decades earlier buffaloes in India were primarily reared for milk production alongwith limited use of mostly males for draught and meat production was a system of utilization of unwanted non-productive animals for which indigenous markets were available. However, during the last two decades buffalo meat production has taken an industrial shape to greater extent and has opened an additional avenue for the profitable rearing of till recently undesired male calves. Due to development of buffalo fattening for export quality meat production, the mortality rate of such calves had shown considerable reduction in the recent years which has been possible only due to better care and management. The purpose of rearing riverine buffaloes are :

1. Milk production
2. Meat production
3. Draught animals

The purpose of rearing swamp buffaloes is although variable but mostly all the three aspects receive equal importance. Unlike swamp buffaloes of other Asian countries in India, selection in swamp buffaloes has also been made for milk production to greater extent as evident from surveys (Pathak and Sikia, 1976; Singh, 1978; Tamuly, 1978).

So far non-descript small sized and relatively thinner buffaloes present in hilly and also in cold region are also reared primarly for milk production and non-productives are used for meat production.

Valuable Byproducts of Buffaloes

In addition to primary products of milk, meat (buffen) and power supply (draught) buffaloes provide different kinds of valuable byproducts. No part of live and dead buffaloes is left unutilized.

1. **Byproducts of live buffaloes:** Dung and urine are produced daily. These are residues of feeds voided after the extraction of nutrients in the gastro intestinal tract. Dung and urine contain nutrients for the herbal crops. The importance of animal droppings is increasing due to increasing demand of herbal foods (foods of plant origin) produced from the use of organic manure. Bovine during is a major source of organic manure in Bharat. Substantial quantity of dung is also made into during cake for fuel.

   Long and coarse hairs of switch of the tail are generally cut at about 6 months interval. Long hairs are used for making ropes and mats etc.

2. **Byproducts of slaughtered buffaloes:** The byproducts of slaughtered buffaloes can be classified into the following categories on the basis of utility.

   a) Byproducts of commercial uses: Hide, horns, hooves and bone are used for leather, feed, manure and omamental product.

   b) Glands like liver, spleen, kidney, genitalia and pituitary etc. are used in pharmaceutical industries.

   c) Blood is used for food and pharmaceutical industries.

3. **Dead animals:** The Carcass of buffaloes not suffering from highly contagious disease is disposed of after flaying for the manufacture of meat meal, bone meal and meat-cum-bone meal. Horns and hooves are used in cottage industry.

4. **Gut contents:** Gut contents, comprising of mostly rumen contents of slaughtered and dead buffaloes, are composed for manure.

Production Systems of Riverine Buffaloes

There is wide variation in the production systems of dairy type riverine buffaloes in India and these are linked with the utility of animals for earning livelihood by low income group and for commercial purpose by the others. A substantial number of medium and large farmers usally keep one or two lactating buffaloes for domestic consumption besides a small number of migratory tribes. Thus, the production systems prevalent in most part of India may be classified as follows:

I. Buffalo production systems in rural areas

Significant improvement has taken place in buffalo production systems of rural areas and this is mostly due to the organization of milk co-operatives and services provided by these co-operatives. Now, awareness about the feeding, breeding and health management of livestock has been considerably increased. The buffalo production system prevalent in rural areas may be further classified as:-

1. **Stall feeding:** This system is followed by the medium and large farmers producing enough dry and green roughages for the feeding or their buffaloes. The main source of dry roughages are wheat straw, jowar kadbi, bajra kadbi in the northern, western and in some central and south states, whereas paddy straw is the staple roughage in most part of Bihar, West Bengal, Orissa dn north-east states. Buffaloes under stall feeding system are fed a reasonably satisfactory diet comprising of a mixture of chaffed straw or stovers, generally cooked slurry of concentrates containing a mixture of crushed cotton seed and/or cotton seed cake, mustard cake (in some ardea groundnut cake or seasame cake or sunflower cake or linseed cake) and often some crushed leguminous seeds like guar, lathyrus and moth etc. and variable quantity of chaffed green fodders. Common cereal green fodders fed in larger part of Indian are jowar, bajra, maize and teosinite during the hot seasons (wet and dry). Berseem, Lucerne, sengi, oats and barely are common green fodders for winter season. Floors, dal chunies and bran are fed through frequent mixing during the feeding time for increasing the intake of diet. This system of feeding is increasing in the milk shed areas where adequate facilities of milk collection and timely money distribution have been made. Farmers in such areas are also using compounded feeds and mineral mixtures for providing a relatively more balanced diet.
2. **Grazing supplemented with stall feeding:** This system is prevalent in states still having large uncultivated land in arid,

semi arid and hilly regions. The buffaloes are allowed 6 to 10 hours grazing daily on the spent and depleted grasslands which generally contains reasonably satisfactory coverable of edible biomass during the wet season but at most of the places these grasslands are highly depleted and inadequate to meet the requirements of grazing buffaloes during lean months of dry seasons which is hot summer in plains and winter in high Himalayan altitudes. The supplement used for the feeding of buffaloes are highly variable and depends on the produciotn stage of buffaloes, marketing facilities and economic status as well as requirement of the owners. In this system, lactating buffaloes are provided concentrates of the owners. In this system, lactating buffaloes are provided concentrates and also green fodder, if available. This is followed by the supplement feeding of working and pregnant buffaloes, Non-productive and non-pregnant dry buffaloes and growing stodk are least cared animals. But female calves receiving better deal. The concentrates fed to buffaloes are area specific but preference is given for the feeding of boiled/ cooked cotton seed and/or cotton seed cake, other oil cakes, wheat bran, rice brand andeoiled rice bran, grain shorting including week seeds, flour cereals grains, broken rice, minor millets and pulses milling byproducts etc. feeding of jaggary, crude molasses and molasses is quite common in the sugarcane producing areas.

Provision of milk collection at a reasobable price and regular payment (daily, weekly or fortnightly) and also facilities for the supply of good quality supplements (concentrate mixture and mineral supplement) at milk collection centres run by milk unions provide more encouragement for the supplemental feeding of buffaloes.

3. **Exclusive grazing:** This system is prevalent smong economically weaker class of landless rural families and migratory families. There is great variation in the buffalo production system on exclusive grazing and so far no authenticated quantitative information is available into the four broad classes.

   a) **Grazing system followed by settled families:** These are mostly landless and economically weaker class of people and mostly without any regular job of permanent nature. Livelyhood is mostly dependent on season employment in agricultural operations and occasional employment in other works. For such families, buffalo rearing is a source of livelihood and subsidiary income and they prefer to keep one or two lactating buffaloes exclusively for the sale of fluid milk. These are mostly joint families where generally aged persons take out animals for grazing on the fallow land, along the canal bunds, road sides, baron land and other such places the ladies and growing children collect grasses (mostly dub) for additional feeding. The families unable to purchase a lactating buffalo go for the rearing of a dry buffalo or growing heifer till the date of calving or last fortnight of preganancy on barter system. In this system, owners give the animals free of cost for rearing and he also bears the risk, whereas families rearing the animals spent on feeding and management. At the terminal stage the valuation of animals is done by a committee of local people agreeable to both parties. The owner of the animal is given first priority for retaining the animal after paying half of the valuated price of the animal otherwise barrower has to pay the same amount for retaining the animal. IF both parties are not interested in keeping the animal, then it is sold and amount recovered is equally distributed between the two parties. In this system, the other party (that rearing the animal) generally receive much less return than the unaccounted input but they do not have any other option for the remunerative utilization of their spare time. The other option for remunerative utilization of their spare time. The other main advantage of buffalo rearing by such families is the availability of dung for fuel which otherwise has to be either purchased or collected by picking small and dry twig from distant places. The dung cake not only meet the domestic need of fuel but also some part is spared for sale that provides money to meet the casual daily needs including procurement of food grains.

b) **Grazing system followed in diara land:** The silt left on either side by rivers after receding of water after rainy season is known as diala land and it is used for the cultivation of vegetable at approachable places and for livestock grazing at distant places. A variety of succulent native dub of thick suckers running partly beneath the sand is quite common on such lands. This is quite nutritious and animals are fed on such landsa for 3-4 montsh during the winter season. The supplement used is mostly a small amount of common salt. This system is prevalent in the doaba areas of north India.

c) Grazing system followed in kutch region: In this are human habitations are at distant places and transportation facilities are not satisfactory. The herds of buffaloes are managed under exclusive grazing system by the members of a group of families. Milk collected in these areas are either made in ghee or sold in towns wherever possible to transport. The buffaloes found in kutch region closely resemble with Murrah and Mehsana breeds but not with Surti, Nili-Ravi or Jaffarabadi breeds.

d) Grazing along water sources and hilly region: This system may be observed in different parts of Madhya Pradesh, Maharashtra, Chattisgarh, Jharkhand and Orissa. Details are not available but during longer period of the year, buffaloes receive inadequate feeds and nutrients which are reflected in their production.

II. Buffalo production system in urban and peri-urban areas

There are well defined systems of buffalo production exclusively for commercial milk production to cater the requirement of fluid milk of thickly populated urban areas. The milk products requirement of urban people is met from the milk supply from rural areas. In urban and peri-urban systems of buffalo production generally there is no consideration of any ethic, social and cultural customs. The animals are only lactating buffaloes with good produciotn potential. The calve are mostly kept neglected which hardly survive more than 30-40 days. After this buffaloes are made to lactate with the help of either of the following methods:

i) Through the feeding of palatable concentrates at the time of milk.

ii) With the help of 'Mahoa' i.e. a straw stuffed dummy of dead calf. This has been found very effective for the buffaloes of "Tarai' breed and often let down may be stimulated in many buffaloes from the same 'mahoa' or 'mahua'.

iii) With the use of oxytocin orposterior pituitary injection.

The size of herds may range from a small group of 10-15 lactating buffaloes to large group of even more thatn 500 lactating buffaloes. Larger groups of 100 to 300 lactating buffaloes are more common in urban and peri-urban localities of big cities and industrial towns. The animals in urban areas get change of movement with the compound from sheds to open feeding stalls and often these animals suffer from lameness of different etiology. Owners prefer to sale out such animal rather than to go for treatment which is mostly uneconomical. In peri-urban areas outing of animal on scrubs is generally allowed for 3 to 6 hours daily due to which their suffering is much less than the urban buffaloes. These animals also get opportunity for wallowing during many months.

In this system, selected buffaloes of high milk production potential are brought from the breeding tract and majority of them disposed of in abattoir after extracting last drop of milk till that is remunerative. The animals are fed on all kinds of purchased feeds due to which non-productive buffaloes are immediately disposed of and abattoirs are easily approachable. Agents of abattoirs also regularly visit to purchase such animals.

Mostly, two systems of feeding and management are followed in this production system:

a) **Exclusive stall feeding:** In this system buffaloes are kept closely tethered on mangers for most of the time. The diet is formed of chaffed straws and stovers mixed with water soaked concentrate mixture and some amount of chaffed green fodder in the 'sani' form. The sani is occasionally turned during feeding and each time a small quantity of ground concentrate (either mixture or brand or floor) is generally sprinkled to increased feed intake. The animals are taken out for milking in morning and evening. The surviving buffalo calves are kept tied around a feeding trough in a corner and in most of the cases offered only the left over of milch buffaloes. These owners usually keep a horse driven cart mainly for the disposal of dung at a predetermined place outside the town . The dung is sold either fresh or after converting into manure or cake. Some owners give dung disposal on contract under barter system. Horse or poney or donkey driven cart is also used for bringing feeds and green fodder form the dealers.

   The animals live in stress condition and occurrence of lameness due to various reasons is quite common. Stall owners prefer to dispose of seriously lame buffaloes rather than to go for treatment. In this system, buffaloes also do not get opportunity for wallowing and they are either washed by water splashing or passing through fountains arranged for washing.

b) **Stall feeding with grazing:** This system of buffalo production is followed mostly in peri-urban area. After morning milking, buffaloes are let loose and driven out on the scrubs around the cities for 3 to 6 hours daily. This provides light exercise and also opportunity for wallowing in a water pool available in the outskits of cities. These water pools are mostly contaminated with the drains opening from the inhibited areas of the cities and often these are sources of pathological organisms. In the water pools of industrial areas contamination of heavy metals is common. However, infestation of most of these water pools with aquatic weeks like water hyacinth, pistia and others are helpful in removing heavy metals, whereas frogs and in certain areas mud tolerant small fishers are helpful in considerable removal of larvae and pupae of mosquitoes.

Concentrated buffalo production system on the stall of urban and peri-urban areas has caused great loss to dairy buffalo resources of this country, Now a days, it is very difficult to get a pure Murrah buffalo and those yielding more than 20 kg milk a day have almost vanished from the buffalo population of this country. Almost same is the fate of Mehsana, Surti and other milch breeds of buffaloes. The loss of valuable germ plasm of outstanding buffaloes of various important dairy breeds will take long time for recuperation.

III. Migratory buffalo production system

Migratory buffalo production systems may be identified in two types:

a) **Well established seasonal migratory system of buffalo production:** This system of buffalo production has been used for centuries for certain tribes settled in the sub-Himalayan forests and their concentration is largest in the forests of Shivalik region. Herd size ranges from 25 to more than 200 buffaloes maintained by the families of variable economic status and manpower. Each herd is constituted of 1 to 5 ponies, equal number of cows and Bhutia, Gaddi or their crossbred dogs. The dogs are kept to guard the camp and protect the animals from the carnivorous wild animals. Migration is seasonal. The animals are grazed in the forests of sub-Himalayan region during the cold months extending from November to March which are shifted to high Himalayan Bugyats or Alpine pasture where they are grazed on the lush growing pastures during the hot months. Generally upward journey to high altitude is started celebrating Holi festival, whereas return journey is scheduled to celebrate

Dipawali at the permanent home in the forest of sub-Himalayan region. The movement of herds is step wise i.e. after traveling for a week herds are comped near local market for few days. The entire journey involves about a fortnight to a month depending on the distance traveled. Each family is fully aware with their area of grazing and any dispute is sorted out by the community Panchayat of elders. Earlier there was problem of liquid milk disposal due to which ghee preparation was the only way of earning. Earlier market of ghee was significantly influenced by the ghee put to sale during April and Maya. This problem has been greatly solved due to availability of suitale motor cycles, availability of petrol and other fuel oil even upto Shri Kedarnath situated at eh height of more than 4500 meters above the mean sea level and establishment of milk collection centres alongwith the roads in high Himalayan villages and twons. This has improved the life style of these tribes and now a days almost all families possess a good transistor and some have also portable televisions. Now larger proportion of fluid milk is being sold either at the milk collection centres or to the Halwais in the town.

b) **Need based migration:** This is followed by nomadic tribes all over the country which are mostly found int eh western, northern and central part. These tribes keep on moving round the year with intermittent camping of generally not more than 5-6 months at a place near a town. However, in certain conditions, camping duration may range from one month to even more than a year. Each family keep few buffaloes, cows, growing heifers, ponies, donkeys, pigs, dogs and chicken and livestock composition may be of one species or mixed species. Grazing and scavenging are the main system of feeding. However, supplemental feeding is not uncommon and quality and quantity of supplements depend on the earning on the day. Animal products are mostly consumed in the family and rarely do they opt for selling some milk, poultry and eggs.

IV. Buffalo production system on hills

Native buffaloes or Himalayan region are smaller in size and lighter in weight. These are kept in small number of 1 to 10 animals for milk production because despite low yielding their milk yield is much higher than the local cows and due to patient grazing behaviour they are able to thrive even on the scanty herbage.

Production system of Swamp Buffaloes

Very little published information is available on the production system of swamp buffaloes. Unlike other countries of swamp buffalo population, the Indian swamp buffaloes have been mostly evolved for milk production and generally males are used for puddling the paddy fields and performing other agricultural operations. The production systems of swamp buffaloes are mostly are specific and limited informations so far available are being presented as follows:

1. Swamp buffalo production system in Assam

Swamp buffalo production system prevalent in different parts of Assam may be described as:

a) Confined management practice followed in lower Assam west to Guwahati city: Mostly less than 10 buffaloes comprising of lactating and dry females, males and followers are kept tethered in thatch sheds or enclosures make of bamboo and three branches. Animals are allowed 6-10 hours grazing and wallowing and also fed on stalls. Lactating buffaloes are fed a cooked concentrate of mustard cake, crushed urad seeds, wheat brand and local rice bran. This practice is also followed on north of the Brahamputra.

b) Production on exclusive grazing along the swamps and forests. This practice is more prevalent in the lower half of the upper Assam i.e. Nowgaon and sibasagar districts. The animals are let loose for grazing and wallowing after milking to morning and then collected herding in the evening. Buffaloes are mostly herded in a bamboo or wooden enclosure. However, calves are provided a thatch shelter (Tamuly, 1978).

c) Production systems in terminal upper Assam of Dibrugatrh and Tinsukia area are mixed type. A mixture of dairy, swamp and their interbred are reared in peri-urban areas on grazing supplemented with sstall feeding. These buffaloes are kept tethered at stall and sheds are also provided, while buffaloes in remote areas are kept on grazing.

d) Swamp buffaloes production in Odisha: Buffaloes in Chilka lake and along other sources are reared on grazing the aquatic and semi-aquatic herbages which are mostly available round the year. This strain of swamp buffalo has high salt tolerance and also capable of grazing while swimming submerged in the water.

In the forest area adjoining Odisha, Madhya Pradesh and Andhra Pradesh, another smaller type capable of grazing on hills and in deep forests are reared on grazing only. The claims about the type of most of buffalo breeds of Orissa are conflicting and it appears that alongwith swamp buffaloes dairy breeds and their intrbreds are also found in the peri-urban ares.

2. Swamp buffalo production system in Odisha and adjoining states

The buffaloes are mostly reared on grazing in swamps, hills, forests, river banks and sea shores. Young calves are normally retained at home upto 5-6 months of age. In some parts calves run with the dams. The grazing animals are generally managed by the young children of 10 to 15 years of age. Buffaloes are normally milked twice, when calves are retained at home only in morning when calves run with dams on the grasslands. Sometimes, intelligent child tames one or two docile buffaloes and suckle their milk direct fromt eh teats.

Chilka buffaloes prefer to graze on submerged plants in the Chilka lake, the buffaloes dive for a short time, collect grass bites beneath the water and them emerge out for chewing and swallowing.

3. Buffalo production in Manipur

Large size black buffaloes are kept tethered in the valley for milk production and small size grey buffaloes are tamed and hunted for meat purpose (Singh, 1978).

Breeding Systems

Two breeding systems followed are:

1. **Natural mating:** In larger population of dairy buffaloes and in almost all swamp buffaloes natural mating is used for breeding. In certain states with better awareness buffalo bulls of mostly known dam's milk yield are used for breeding. But, in most part there is no consideration of pedigree and any potent entire male available at estrus is used for breeding. This practice has caused great deterioration in the performance of buffaloes and the destruction of breed characteristic.
2. **Artificial insemination:** Both fresh or short duration stored extended liquid semen as well as frozen semen is being used for the insemination of buffaloes. The service is being provided on

nominal payment by the state department of Veterinary and Animal husbandry and other agencies like BAIF and NDDB. Network project on buffalo development of ICAR is specially arranging breeding with the use of frozen semen of known pedigree and in this programme Murrah, Nili-Ravi, Surti, Bhadawari, Pandharpuri and swamp buffaloes of Assam have been included at present.

Application of embryo transfer technology is still limited to research institutions and my take some more time even for the multiplication of elite animals of very higher production potential.

Problems Associated with Breeding

Although concentration of all good breeds of dairy type river buffaloes is greater in the hot and hot humid parts of tropical India, but problem of low fertility in summer is also more serious in buffaloes than the cattle. Some of the main reproductive problems of economic importance may be enumerated as follows:

1. **Delayed maturity:** Delayed maturity both in male and female buffaloes is common throughout the country. This is due to neglect of calves during growing period. Buffaloes have a potential to gain at the rate of 400 to 800 g daily after 4-6 months of age and can attain 300 to 450 kg body weight suitable for breeding at about 24 months of age (Ranjhan and Pathak, 1999; Mandal *et al.*, 2002), but in majority of dairy buffaloes calving occurs at 4 to 6 years of age. This is mostly due to inadequate supply of feeds and nutrients during the growing phase (Ranjhan and Pathak, 1992).

2. **High incidence of silent oestrus and short duration oestrus:** This is more serious problem during hot and humid-hot months. Due to these reasons often heat is missed and tethered females or females grazing without a potent male in the herd remain unbred. This is one of the important factors besides many others for long intercalving period.

3. **Non-availability of proven sire and good quality semen of proven buffalo bulls:** There is great shortage of potent bulls of known pedigree and production of good quality frozen semen in highly insufficient due to non-availability of required number of the buffalo bulls of desired traits.

4. **Occurrence of venereal diseases causing infertility and sterility:** These problems are encountered in both sexes and cause of spread is the use of bulls for natural service. In recent years these problems are apparently showing an increasing pattern and probably it is due to increased use of artificial insemination in remote villages with the help of improperly trained inseminators which have been provided part time casual employment. In many parts such persons have started projecting themselves as a veterinary doctor and most of them have started veterinary practice without any education and training for handling clinical cases. This is going to be another serous problem in health management of livestock and instead of doing good these half baked personnel may cause more damage to livestock wealth of the country.

Buffaloes are slaughtered for meat production since epic period in India in the name to religious rituals or otherwise (Pathak, 2001). However, during last century buffaloes disposed of for meat production were mostly retired males, aged and weight were rarely available for meat production because buffalo male calves were the most neglected among all the domesticated animals of the indian farmers. However, a fattening study of long duration carried on poor and retarded male buffalo calves of 8 to 12 montsh of age and 60 to 100 kg body weight clearly demonstrated the inherent growth potential when daily gain in body weight obtained was 400 to 700 g and buffloes yielded very good edible carcass at 300 to 350 kg body weight and about 24-30 months of age (Agarwal, 1974). This was followed by a series of studies in the Animal Nutrition Division at the Indian Veterinary Research Institute, Izatnagar (Pathak 1984; Pathak *et al.*,. 1987; Baruah *et al.*,., 1982, 1987). The information on buffalo fattening has been compiled in the formk of a bulletin (Pathka, 1997). Later on more fattening studies conducted at NDRI, Karnal and CIRB, Sub-campus Nabha recorded similar results. Encouraged by these results, now a few reputed parties have entered in the buffalo fattening business and Hind Agro, New Delhi has involved farmers in the programme, which has been found to be remunerative for the farmers. This has also saved many a young calves from premature death through the cruel act of wanton starvation.

Buffalo Dung

It is used as manure and fuel, Had there not been bovine dung in the rural areas, it would have been very difficult to cook food and also combat the cold waves of winter season when temperature falls below 5°C during December-January in most part of the northern India and most of the families do not have enough clothes and bedding for protecting them. Dung mixed with clay is also used for plastering walls made of mud and floor of the house.

Status of Scientific Information on Bhartiya (Indian) Buffaloes

Despite significant contributions in food production and economics of Indian farmers, the buffaloes remained neglected for longer period by the scientific community. This caused great deterioration in the production potential of famous dairy type riverine breeds of northern and western India, due to lifting of high milk producing animals from breeding tract to big cities exclusively for commercial purpose. Milk was extracted to last drop through the use of hormones, calves were made to die in early age of 3-6 weeks and at the end of lactation these valuable germplasm were finally disposed of in slaughter houses.

1. Types and breeds of buffaloes

In India still there are scattered small herds of wild buffaloes, but probably there is no information about the genetic make up of wild buffaloes and relationship between different herds of wild buffaloes with domesticated buffaloes. Long dairy back Indian domesticated dairy buffaloes were distinguished into several breeds ranging from Murrah to Jarangi (Littlewood, 1936; Oliver 1938; Naryan Reddi, 1939; ICAR, 1939; Dave, 1940; Kaura, 1952; ICAR, 1960). However, in all these publications there appears to be no authentic statement on the swamp buffaloes, which was later mentioned by Mc Gregor (141) in his extensive work bmbodied in his doctorate thesis. In later publications emphasis has been given only on limited dairy type riverine breeds and even tody status of the buffaloes of Himalayan states, states of north-eastern hill region and large areas of Orissa, Jharkhand, Madhya Pradesh and Andhra Pradesh possessing different kinds of buffloes is not fully known. More than 6 breeds of buffaloes have been mentioned in Orissa along (Samal, 1988) and two types each in Assam (Tamuly, 1978) and Manipur (Singh, 1978).

Thus, there is urgent need of typing and characterization of all types of buffaloes found in India. It is not a easy job and required concerted efforts. While typing and characterizing the buffaloes it is also important to involve such local people which are actually involved in the rearing of buffaloes for several generations. So far it is believed on the basis of several statements that milk yield of swamp buffaloes is very low, but observations in native buffaloes are the yield of 1.8 to 3.11 kg average daily yield in Assamese swamp buffaloes (Tamuly, 1978) to 610 to 1277 kg milk production during 206 to 274 days lactation length in swamp buffloes of Manipur, recorded in 4th lactation of some animals (Singh, 1978). These two studies themselves are the indicators of inadequate information about the swamp buffaloes. Probably no such detailed informations are available about the buffaloes of Orissa, high Himalayan states and Andaman and Nicobar islands. In generalized statement 1-2 litres milk yield in Manda and Kalahandi buffaloes 2-3 litres in Sambalpuri and Dhenkanal type, 4 kg in Kujang type and 3-4 litres in large size Paralakemedi buffaloes. So far, probably no estimate is available about the milk yield of Bheda and Parikud buffaloes thriving in saline water areas of coastal regions of Orissa (Samal, 1988).

2. Feeds, nutrition and feeding

During the last three decades considerable information has been generated on the nutrition and feeding of buffaloes during different physiological states of most of dairy type riverine buffaloes, which have helped in evolving a satisfactory feeding standard (Mandal *et al.*, 2002). However, there is need of long term feeding trails on adequate feeding for establishing the optimum production potential in terms of milk, milk fat, meat and power for different breeds of river as well as swamp type buffaloes.

The research works in the search and utilization of non-conventional feeds for more than half a century have yielded mostly non-conclusive results and least adaptable technologies. The time has come to realize that for extraction of inherent production potential, it is necessary to provide the required amount of nutrients through the feeding of palatable feeds. Thus, all research project funded from public resources should be reoriented for evolving optimum feeding systems to take maximum advantage from the buffaloes through the support of management and health care. Information so far generated for the nutritional improvement of low grade cereal crop residues and other non-conventional feeds may be utilized for the feeding of large population of low producing the non-productive surplus cattle which has no avenue for disposal. Further, other non-conventional feeds shuld be restricted to very specific and well defined projects considering economic viability. Now researches on the development of balanced diets suitable for sustaining the inherent productivity of buffaloes under variable climatic conditions is more important. It should be further supported by the technological and biotechnological approaches for increasing the efficiency of nutrients utilization by reducing the losses (particularly that of energy) through various unwanted products of fermentation as well as altering the ratio of volatile fatty acids. Due to intensive cropping, depletion of micro minerals is very high and it is becoming the cause of many deficiency problems. Most of such deficiencies at subclinical level have adverse effect on the productivity of the animals. Therefore, emphasis should be given for further studies on such aspects.

3. Management of buffaloes

Three main constraints are important in the management of buffaloes. These are (i) summer stress, (ii) winter stress at high altitude and (iii) inadequate availability of non-polluted wholesome water for drinking and wallowing. The problem of water supply is becoming serious every day and it requires special attention of state for the maintenance of riverine buffaloes, one of the most important dairy animals of the twenty first century.

If we look back on the availability of wholesome water, it was plenty in this country and about three decades earlier it was a common scene to see herds of buffaloes enjoying wallowing in different rivers, streams, lakes and ponds. But now a days a large number of urban and peri-urban agglomeration of buffaloes are seen lying in the dirty and polluted muddy waters around the cities and in the waters polluted with industrial affluent along the industrial township. Even large rivers like Ganga, Yamuna, Narmada, Krishna, KIaveri etc. are also unable to contain enough water for several montsh due to many man made obstructions. Most of these rivers are also polluted by the drainage of urban garbage and industrial affluent as well as disposal of dead bodies in many areas as availability of fuel for funeral is decreasing as well its cost is increasing.

Therefore, there is urgent need for making arrangements for the supply of enough wholesome water for drinking and wallowing in rural areas. The later can be compensated with arrangements of shower bath in th urban and peri-urban areas where owners keep more than 50 lactating buffaloes crowded in a limited space. Since most of the waters are polluted and infected, there is need for the arrangements of better hygienic conditions for reducing morbidity and other losses due to sub-clinical infections and infestations.

Maintenance of hygienic conditions in buffalo farms and dairy buffalo staffs is much less expensive. Provision of dry place for resting, timely disposal of dung and urine, daily washing/wallowing, sprinking of phelyl lotions in water, occasional application of flaked lime powder and use of gunny bags soaked in saturated solution of washing soda at the entrance particularly during the spread of viral diseases like foot and mouth disease may be considered useful for providing reasonably satisfactory protection against may diseases.

4. Health care

Health problems of buffaloes may be widespread or localized (Pathak and Sharma, 1988). There is need of seasonal protective vaccinations agains thaemorrhagic septicemia, foot and mouth diseas and in some area also balck quarter. Vacchines are available but farmers often complain for the effectiveness of vaccinations particularly the protection provided by broth vaccine for HS and use of oil adjuvant vaccine frequently leaves behind a tumerous growth which subsides after a long time. Adequate coverage against parasitism is necessary to minimize the losses caused by morbidity and mortality. Early life or even pre-nata infestation to Toxocara vitulorum (Neoascaris vitulorum) is responsible for large number of death of cavles not only in India but also in many other countries. This can be easily prevented to a greater extent by using deworming in the first of fourth week of life, which can be further repeated, if necessary. Coccidiosis is another serios problem in young calves below six montsh of age when roughages in their diet is a less. There is a long list of diseases but at the same time the list of limited bacterial, viral, parasitic and nutrition-metabolic diseases need special attention of states. There is need of buffalo owners about the economic effect of these disease, methods of protecting the animals and follow up action. The list of such disease, place of availability of vaccines and drugs and place of assistance for providing veterinary services should be prominently displayed at public institutions like veterinary hospitals, Panchayat Bhavan, Cooperative stores, block office and village school etc. Services of local channels of radio and television should also be made available for educating the livestock owners. Livestock husbandry specially buffalo keeping is increasing its commercial dimension and development of buffalo meat production has opened new avenue for the fattening of so far neglected male calves for good quality meat production.

Employment Potential of Buffalo Production

Buffalo production systems in vogue have provided a large number of part time and full time employment, which are supplementary as well as sustaining. The prevalent system of keeping a few lactating buffaloes has also provided employment to such persons who are not able to get employment even for relatively lighter obs. Different kinds of employment associated with present systems of buffalo production may be classified as follows:

1. **Part time employment:** Larger number of families and people are involved. In this system, only a few number 91-5) of lactating buffaloes and their young calves (if survive the neglect) are kept for selling liquid milk and part of dung after making dung cake. Some amount of composted dung is either used or sold as manure. Generally aged family members, ladies and young children are engaged in feeding, watering, washing, grazing, milk and marketing of milk etc. Labour put for these works by the family members is not accounted. Any accounting of these inputs will make the milk production non-remunerative at the present marketing rates. Since major of these persons do not have any remunerative engagement, they do not have any other option but to opt for animal husbandry.

2. **Employment for grazing:** In areas where fallow and wasteland is available, some people opt for grazing against payment which may be cash or kind. In morning buffaloes are collected and returned safe in evening. Grazing of buffaloes also including wallowing.

3. **Employment for milking:** This is mostly a part time but regular job without any holiday. Professional milkers are generally engaged by non-farming communities which mostly keep one lactating buffalo or cow for milk and milk products for domestic consumption.

4. **Employment for cleaning and dung disposal:** This is also part time job mostly on barter system. The persons evolved clean the

shed, collect dung and prepare dung cake which is equally shared by the employer and employee.

5. **Milk collection and disposal:** This job is common around the towns, cities and industrial township. People engaged in this job collect milk from door to door for sale mostly at fixed shops daily. Payment is made daily or weekly. Sometime advance is also paid and in such cases producers are paid less price than the regular rates.

6. **Employment in milk processing and products making:** This is highly variable and may be organized or unorganized sector. The agencies involved in processing and products making of milk are:

   i) Sweet meat makers or Halwais

   ii) Milk processing plants: The products generally whole milk, standardized milk, toned milk, double toned milk, paneer, cheese, cream, buttern and ghee

   iii) Ice cream factories

   The whole production and marketing systems provide large number of employment at various levels right from collection of milk to sale of products passing through processing, packaging, storage and transportation etc.

7. **Employment in meat production:** Similarly meat production industries may be either (i) small for locak consumers or (ii) large for export and /or further processing for the preparation of meat products. Retail sale of meat and meat products also provide employment.

8. Employment in Carcass disposal:

   i) Leather industry

   ii) Leather goods industry

   iii) Meat meal industry

   iv) Bone Processing industry

      a) Glue

      b) Gelatin

      c) Fat

d)Other industrial oil

e) Pharmaceutical products from glands

f) Meat meal, bone meal etc.

9. Marketing of buffaloes:

i) Door to Door in the breeding tract

ii) Weekly, fortnightly and monthly markets

iii)Seasonal animal fairs mostly organized on some occasions. These are large fairs lasting for one week to 30 days at six montly or annual interval.

Further Research Requirements

During past three-four decades extensive research works have been done on various aspects of buffalo production but three appears to be lack of coordination and series gap in the exchange of knowledge gained at different centres. If timely action will not be taken, other countries may be leader in buffalo production utilizing the Indian germplasm resources. Thus, there is need of serious thoughts for the reorlentation of research projects on various aspects of buffalo production and its coordination and monitoring. The important areas may be demarcated as:

1. **Classification, breeding and reproduction:**

i) All types of buffaloes need characterization for qualitative and quantitative traits.

ii) There is urgent need of the production of progeny tested bulls, at least of those breeds which are in international demand.

iii)Development and refinement of technologies for the production of international grade frozen semen. This has a great international market.

iv)Conservation of all native germ plasm of buffaloes (domesticated and wild) in situ.

2. **Nutrition and feeding:** Areas of research requiring more attention are:

i) The development of complete ration for supporting (a) moderate growth for the production of replacement stock i.e.

buffalo heifers of 400±50 kg body weight of large breeds and 300±20 kg body weight in medium sized breeds at two years of age, and bulls of 500 and 400 kg body weights of respective types at about 30 months of age. Larger number of residual male buffalo calves may be divided into two classes as per requirements for the purpose of feeding. Rearing of male calves for the production of working animals required a diet to supply a growth for attaining about 300 to 400 kg body weight at about 3 years of age, which provides adequate time for the development of strong bones, particularly limb bones and ligamentum nuche. The other group of male calves will need high energy-high protein diets to supply 600 to 800 g daily gain in body weight so that good quality buffalo meat could be produced by sacrificing the animals of 300 to 350 kg body weight at 12-15 months of age.

ii) Development of diets for supporting optimum milk production while maintaining the normal reproduction.

iii) Development of harmless additives for enhancing nutrients utiliztion by educing wasteful losses.

3. **Health Management:** The areas of research requiring priority may be :

i) Further refinement of available vaccines partucarly against HS and FMD infections.

ii) Development of vaccines against the emerging microbial diseases.

iii) Development of measures for providing protection against haemoprotozoan and enteric protozoal infection.

iv) Development of package of practice for protein against helminthes and octoparasites.

Future of Buffaloes

It is very bright and buffaloes are emerging as the food animal of the twenty first century due to many factors like:

1. High adaptability of the animals in widely variable agro-climatic conditions.
2. Comparatively less selective and capable of handling greater proportion of roughages in diet.

3. Carcass is much leaner and cholesterol content is very low.
4. Amino acid composition of flesh is much balanced than most of the edible meats of other species.
5. Horsing and management is much easier.
6. They have reasonable disease resistance.

References

Acharya, R.M. 1991. Proceeding of Third World Buffalo Congress, Bulgaria, May 13-18.

Adlakha, S.C. and Sharma, S.N. 1992. Diseases. *In:* Buffalo Production. Elsevier. The Netherlands.

Agarwal, V.P. 1974. Doctorate research carried at IVRI, Izatnagar. Agra University, Agra.

Bhat, P.N. 1992. Genetics of river bufafloes. *In :* Buffalo Production. World Animal Series. Elsevier. The Neitherlands.

Bhatia, B.B. 1992. Parasitism of river buffaloes. *In:* Buffalo Production. World Animal Series, Elsevier. The Netherlands.

Baruah, K.K., Ranjhan, S.K. and Pathak, N.N. 1982. Effect of various levels of protein and energy feeding on growth, digestibility of organic nutrients and carcass characteristics of Indian desi male buffalo calves. Proc. 2nd Asian-Astralasian Assoc. Anim. Prod. Soc., PICC, Manila. November 10-13.

Baruah, K.K., Ranjhan, S.K. and Pathak, N.N. 1987. Growth response, feed efficiency and carcass characteristics of Indian buffalo (*Bubalus bubalis*) calves fattened on different plane of nutrition. Buffalo Bulletin, 8:77.

Cockrill, W.R. 1974. The Husbandry and Health of the Domestic Buffalo, FAO, Rome.

Dave, C.N. 1940. Pooma Agric. College Magazine, 32:97.

Gupta, B.N., Murty, V.N., Khan, S.A. and Mishra, B.P. 1968. Indian Vet. J., 45: 858.

ICAR 1985. Nutrient Requirements of Livestock and Poultry, ICAR, New Delhi.

Kaura, R.L. 1952. Indian Breeds of Livestock (including Pakistan). Prem. Publishers, Lucknow.

Kearl, L.C. 1982. Nutrients Requiremetns of Ruminants in Developing Countries. Utah State University, Logo, Utah, USA.

Kamra, D.N. 2002. Personal communication.

Littlewood, R.W. 1936. Livestock of Sourthern India, Government Press, Madras.

Mandal, A.B., Paul, S.S. and Pthak, N.N. 2002. Nutrient requirements and Feeding of Buffaloes and Cattle. International Book Publishing House, Charbagh, Lucknow.

Meson, I.L., 1969. A World Dictionary of Livestock Breeds and Types. CAB Technical Comm., England.

McGregor, 1941. Thesis of buffalo. Royal Veterinary College, London.

Narayana Reddi, M.L. 1929. Madras Agric J., 27:50.

Negi, S.S., Joshi, B.C. and Kehar, N.D. 1968. Punjab Agril., Univ. J. Res. 5:92.

Oliver, A. 1938. A Brief survey of some of the important breeds of cattle in India. ICAR Bulletin No. 17, New Delhi.

Pathak, N.N. 1985. Proc. National Symp. On the use of Nuclear Technique in Animal Health and Production. IVRI, Izatnagar, April, 4-6.

Pathak, N.N. 1988. Feeding Standard or Buffaloes. Animal Nutrition Division Publication, IVRI, Izatnagar.

Ptahak, N.N. 1996. Nutrition and feeding of male buffalo calves for the production of meat and working animals. Pub., No. 34. IVRI, Izatnagar.

Pathak, N.N. 2001. A guide for feeding of dairy buffaloes. CIRB, Hisar.

Pathak, N.N. and Sharma, M.C. 1988. Health management of buffalo. *In :* Buffalo Production. II World Buffalo Congress. New Delhi.

Pathak, N.N. and Verma, D.N. 1993. Nutrient Requirements of Buffalo. International Book Dist. Co., Lucknow.

Pathak, N.N., Ranjhan, S.K. and Baruah, K.K. 1987. Growth response, feed efficiency and carcass characteristics of Indian buffalo calves (*Bubalus bubalis*) fattened on different plane of nutrition, Buffalo Bulletin, 8:77.

Pathak, N.N. and Saikia, A., 1976. Final Report of Animal Nutrition Survey in Assam, Veterinary College, Khanapara, Guwahati.

Ranjhan, S.K. 1998. Nutrient requirement and Feeding of Farm animals. ICAR, New Delhi.

Ranjhan, S.K. and Pathak, N.N. 1989. Feeding and Management of Buffaloes. Vikas Pub., House, Pvt. Ltd., New Delhi.

Ranjhan, S.K. and Pathak, N.N. 1993. Text book on Buffalo Production. 3rd edn. Vikas Pub. House Pvt. Ltd., New Delhi.

Ranjhan, S.K. and Pathak, N.N. 1999. Text Book on Buffalo Production. 4th edn. Vikas Pub., House Pvt. Ltd., New Delhi.

Samal, B. 1988. A Short History of Veterinary Medicine and Animal Husbandry in Orissa. Puspagiri Press, Cuttack, Orissa.

Sen, K.C., Ray, S.N. and Ranjhan, S.K. 1978. Nutrient Requirements and Feeding of Farm Animals. ICAR, New Delhi.

Singh, D. 1978. Studies on Certain Economic Traits of Indigenous Buffalo of Manipur. M.V.Sc. Thesis. Assam Agricultural University, Khanapara, Guwahati.

Tamul, B.C. 1978. Studies on Certain Physical Characteristics and Production Performances of Swamp Buffalo of Assam. M.V.Sc. Thesis. Assam Agricultural University, Khanapara, Guwahati.

❑❑❑

3

Mammary Gland and Lactation

Introduction

Like other ruminant mammalians buffalo possesses mammary gland (udder) in the inguinal region. It is a modified cutaneous gland for highly specific function of milk production, which is the natural food of new born calves. The cellular differentiation of the mammary glands occurs in the early pre-natal stage from the dermal cell on the ventral surface of embryos in the inguinal region. During the process of foetal development, these mammary cells aggregate to form four distinct mammary buds, that is two on either side of the mid line. The formation of gland is almost similar in both sexes except that the development of teats in p[re-natal growth is much slow in male foetus. The development of non-glandular portion consisting of connective tissue and fat pads almost complete by the time of birth. Apparently there is little difference in the teats of male and female calves at birth. Active development of mammary glands takes place in the early post-natal life at a much higher rate than the overall body growth. Larger portion of mammary ducts row before conception and the formation of alveoli starts with the conception with gradually replace the pad of the fat tissue of the udder. Normally secretion of life starts immediately after the birth of calf but in exceptionally high yielding females it may start a few days earlier than the calving date.

Anatomy of the Udder

The mammary glands are collectively known as udder. Buffalo udder contains four mammary glands situated two on either side parallel to mid line in the inguinal region. The two lateral halves of udder have clear external demarcation at the side of median suspensary ligament, which is distinct when viewed from the rear. The front attachment of udder is with abdominal wall and ear is folded with high between the two hind limbs. The udder of dairy type riverine buffaloes is much large and voluminous than the drought type swamp buffaloes and their wild ancestors. The four quarters of udder of dairy buffaloes should be well developed and almost similar in shape and size of convenient milking particularly for the use of machine milking. The length, width and girth of udder and udder score, and type of udder significantly affect the milk yield (Taneja and BHatnagar, 1958; Saxena and Prabhu, 1970; Saxena, 1973; Saakova, 1979; Turabov and Abullaev, 1979; Hafeez and Naidu, 1981; Tsankova, 1983). Usually fore quarters are less voluminous with smaller tears than the rear quarters and yielding significantly less milk (Polikhronov and Tosev, 1970; Ragab *et al.*, 11971; Tsankova and Tosev, 1980; Pandey *et al.*, 1981; Alim *et al.*, 1982; Tripathi and Saraswat, 1982). Normally there is an increase in length, width and overall score of udder upto third lactation after that there was decrease in milk yield during the subsequent lactation but udder characteristics remained almost unchanged (Hafeez and Naidu, 1981).

In the process of milking or suckling by the calf the milk flows out of the mammary glands through the teat canal. In buffaloes front teats are shorter and thinner than the rear tears (Saakova, 1979b). Supernumerary leats are often present length and important reproductive traints (Dwivedi and Prabhu, 1970; Ludri and Sarma, 1981; Verma *et al.*, 1984). An exceptional instance of the fusion of left fore and rear teats and another specimen with five functional teats has been reported in swamp buffalo (Fischer, 1962).

Parts of the Udder

The udder consists of external and internal supporting structures, circulatory vessels, lymph vessels and glandular parenchyma with lacteal canals opening into the cistern. All parts of udder play important role in the milk production.

Skin

The skin of udder is thinner than the body and encapsulates the mammary glands. Besides providing support it protects glands from the external injuries and invasion of microorganisms. The skin is connected with the mammary glands with a sheet of fine connective tissue, and fore quarters are connected with abdomen with a coarse connective tissue

Suspensory apparatus

The suspensory apparatus of the udder is formed from the two layers of lateral and two layers of median suspensory ligaments (Katiyar and Chandra, 1983). The suspensory ligaments are the most important supporting components of the udder.

a) **Lateral suspensory ligaments:** The two layers of lateral suspensory ligaments are present on either side of the udder. They emerge from the sub-pelvic and republic tendons. Immediately after origin the lateral suspensory ligament I divided into a thin superficial and thick deeper sheets. The superficial part is attached to semimembranous and abductor muscles. The thicker part is larger than the thinner superficial part and extended downward and forward covering the convex lateral surface of udder and large number of lamellae from the thicker part penetrate in interior of the glands forming composed of elastic and collagenous fibvres of connective tissue.The fibres are mostly arranged longitudinally and transverse; and oblique arrangements are rarely found. The elastic fibres are thicker in outer and middle and thinner in the linner zone of the lateral suspensory ligament (Katiyar and Chandra, 1983).

b) **Median suspensory ligaments:** These ligaments are the main supporting tissue of the udder. They extend between he right and left halves of the udder and these are separated from eath other after some gap from their origin. The median suspensory ligaments are formed byt eh reflection of the two lamellae of the yellow elastic fibres originated from the abdominal tunic at some distance posterior to the umbilicus and have firm attachment with the mid line near the centre of gravity of the udder. Posteriorly they extend near to the ischial arch. These ligaments are mainly composed of elastic fibres which are thicker than the fibres of the lateral suspensory ligaments.

The fibres arrangement is oblique and transverse int eh outer and inner zone, and longitudinal in the middle zone

Numerous lamellae of median suspensory ligaments extend into the gland parenchyma and form sling-like supporting arrangements by joining with the lamellae of the lateral suspensory ligaments. In addition to suspensory ligaments the abdominal tunic is also attached firmly on the dorsal concave surface of the mammary glands of buffalo.

Vascular system

The largest volume of oxygenated blood from heart is supplied to the mammary glands by paired external pudic arteries arising from the posterior aorta in the inguinal region (Hossain *et al.,* 1980; Bhadawai *et al.,*. 1985). The other sources of blood supply are the right and left common iliac artries and the external iliac arteries. The external pudic arteries emerge through the external inguinal ring and then extend as the mammary arteries. Great variation may be seen in the branching pattern of the mammary artery between the animals. The branching is more in high milk yielding buffaloes. Just after entering the udder the mammary artery of each lateral half is divided into two main branches, the cranial mammary artery and the caudal mammary artery. In large size udders of heavy milk yielders, two additional off shoots of caudal mammary artery are given off before the origin of the main caudal mammary artery. The additional caudal mammary arteries of almost equal diameter to that of main caudal mammary artery branch extensively and supply the posterior part of the udder.

Cow like pattern of branching of mammary artery is also observed in many buffaloes. In such cases, the cranial branch of the mammary artery travels about two third of the gland then bifurcates into the cranial mammary artery supply to fore that and udder. The main trunk extends forward as subcutaneous abdominal artery and terminates in front of the base of udder (Katiyar and Chandra, 1983).

a) **Cranial mammary artery:** The cranial mammary artery extends forward the brancing of caudal mammary artery. It runs cranio-ventrally, continues distally and terminates ont eh cranio-lateral aspects of the fore teat as papillary artery. In its course numerous small branches arise and enter into the fore quarter of the udder.

b) **Caudal mammary artery:** It travels almost ventrally in the hind quarter of udder form an arch. The convexity of caudal mammary artery is directed cranial. The ventral course gives rise to a large branch extending downward and forward in the glandular parenchyma of the hind quarter of udder and finally terminates in the lateral wall of the rear teat The posterior branch of the caudal mammary artery ramifies in the posterior part of the mammary gland.

Anastomoses between the capillaries of the cranial mammary artery and the cranial branch of the caudal mammary artery and also between the final vessels of the two halves of udder occur in buffaloes (Hossain *et al.*, 1980; Katiyar and Chandra, 1983).

c) **Subcutaneous abdominal artery:** In many buffaloes, the subcutaneous artery an extension after the branding of the cranial mammary artery. It runs cranially in the glandular tissue near the lateral basal border and ramifies in ventral abdominal wall in front of the base of the udder. Several lateral, medial and ventral branches of subcutaneous abdominal artery supply the glandular mammary tissues.

d) **Perineal artery:** A branch of posterior aorta at the ventral commissure of the vulva is called perineal artery, which extends ventrocranial under the skin in the perineal region. Near the caudoventral region of the mammary gland several branches emerge to supply the mammary fascia of the rear quarters. Usually no branch extends into the mammary gland.

The supra-mammary lymph glands are supplied by a thin branch of the mammary artery, which emerges before its bifurcation into the cranial and caudal branches. The vessels are more large and tortuous in the voluminous udder of high milk production buffaloes.

The intermediate layer of the wall of teats is the vessels zone of an extensive network of blood vessels. In the teats of the virgin heifers the artiries are almost straight and muscular. The arteries supplying lactating teats are highly thickened and tortuous in their course due to an increase in fibro-muscular tissues around them. The blood low of teat arteries is controlled by valves like arterial bolsters of various types (Moussa, 1982).

At the point of termination of capillaries origin of venules takes place which subsequently anastomose with each other to form the mammary veins that drain blood from the udder. The veins of udder transverse almost adjoining with the mammary arterial system. The blood flows through the external pudic veins, external veins and perineal veins into the posterior vena cava.

The second channel for the return of blood comprises of two subcutaneous abdominal veins commonly known as milk veins. These emerge at the anterior border of the udder. The flow of blood is directed towards of udder in the region posterior to the umbilicus in young animals. The valve of veins become ineffective in lactating animals and can flow either way, that is towards anterior vena cava as well as the udder.

An increase in blood flow towards the udder and decrease in uterine circulation is observed during the early post-partum period. This probably plays an important role in the initiation of milk secretion by the increased flow of milk precursors and lactogenic hormones into the mammary glands. The flow rate of blood towards the udder continues to rise upto the peak yield period and thereafter starts gradual decline. The flow rate of blood in the udder is none of the most important factor the regulating the milk production in the lactating animals.

e) **Lymphatic system:** The lymph is a colourless body fluid originating from the filtration of blood and its composition is similar to the blood except that the lymph is devoid of blood cells and contains lower concentration of protein. The exchange between the constituents of blood plasma and interstitial fluid largely contrigubtes in the production of lymph. The mammary glands are transverse by an extensive proliferation of lymph vessels. The mammary glands are drained by the superficial and deep set of lymph channels. The superficial vessels are spread all around the surface of the mammary glands beneath the cover of skin, fascia and a thick layer of adipose tissues. Some of the superficial lymphatics transverse through the layer of adipose tissue, while majority are in direct contact with the glandular parenchyma. Anastomoses occur between the lymphatics of the fore and rear quarters of the same side but not with the other side. This plays significant role in controlling the infections from one side to other side. Many minor superficial lymphatics arise from the glandular parenchyma at the ventral border of the mammary gland and around the base of the teats. They move tortuously upwards on the lateral surface of the body of mammary glands (corpus mammae). In their course some of the lymph vessels receive dorsally the lumphatics draining the grandular parenchyma. All these lymph canals terminate at different vessels on the ventral border on the supramammary lymph node.

Some of the lymph vessels arising from the cranial quarter merge with the vessels of the caudal quarter of the same side and vice versa. Other lymphatics of the cranial quarter ramify on the lateral surface of the mammary gland, move caudal and terminate at the cranial border of the mammary lymph node.

The lymphatics on the caudal surface of the mammary glands ran a tortuous course dorsally and cranially and terminate as the afferent ducts of the mammary lymph node. The other unite with the lymphatics of the lateral surface and then terminate on the ventral border of the mammary lymph gland. The lymph vessels of the mammary septa and the base of the mammary gland terminated on the medial surface of the mammary lymph node. The deep parenchyma of mammary glands was drained either directly or coalesced with the superficial lymphatics into the mammary lymph gland. The mammary lymph glands (nodes) are two in number situated on either side of the mid line near the caudal aspect of the base of the udder beneath the thick layer of adipose tissue. A notch on the dorsal border of mammary lymph bland represents the hilus. The mammary lymph nodes are flattened and oval or somewhat triangular in shape. The length ranged from 5 to 7 cm and width form 3 to 5.5 cm.

The efferent lymph vessels of the mammary lymph nodes are 6-7 in number of which 2-3 vessels of cranial group after arising from the hilus ran cranio-dorsally in a tortuous fashion and cross the mammary vessels. After this they run dorsally to enter the inguinal canal along the cranial border of the external pudic veins beneath the cover of external oblique muscle of the abdomen. Thes lymphatcis then cross the vein near near the ventral aspects of the body of ilium to turn abruptly posterior and ventral to enter into the iliofemoral lymph node. The caudal groups of efferent lymph vesels are bigger in diameter and more tortuous than the cranial group. After leaving the hilus of the lymph node they move dorsally and enter the inguinal canal, where they extent posterior to the external pudic artery for a short distance and cross it beneath the ilium before termination at the lateral surface of the iliofemoral lymph node, also known as deep inguinal lymph gland. This gland is situated under the body of ilium in the angle formed by the external iliac and circumflex iliac arteries. Its shape is oval, length ranges from 7-9.9 cm and width 4-7 cm (Barnwal and Dhingra, 1978).

Nerve Supply

The mammary glands are supplied with afferent (sensory) and efferent (motor) nerves of the sympathetic nerve fibres. These nerves arise from the ventral lumbar, inguinal and perineal branches. The sensory nerves are important in the milk-ejection mechanism. The motor nerves regulate blood supply and innervate The smooth muscles around the milk collecting ducts and the teat sphincter. Since nerves of the mammary glands are in the connective tissue and not in direct contact with the alveolar cells of the parenchyma, there seems to be no direct effect of nerve supply on the rate of secretion and composition of milk of milk. Excitement stimulates the secretion of the hormone epinephrine, which has vasoconstriction property and has inhibitory effect on the milk secretion. Massage, temperature and suckling of teats stimulate the secretion of oxytocin form the pituitary gland, which reduces let down of milk.

Mammary duct system

A series of ductules draining from the alveoli through larger channels into the teat cistern and ending at the steam canal form the mammary the mammary duct system. The ductules and secretory lobules are supported by intralobular and interlobular connective tissue speta. The quantity of the connective tissue is more in low milk producing animals, whereas mammary glands of high milk producing buffaloes contain larger proportion of alveolar tissue and ductular tissue with minimum around of connective tissue. In Egyptian buffaloes the ratio between glandular and non-glandular tissues of heavy yielders has been reported to be 1.79, which is almost double than the 0.82 observed in the low milk yielders (Nosier, 1972). The opening of streak canal of the teats is controlled by strong sphincter muscles and streak canal is the continuation of the team cistern. The teat cistern continues as the gland cistern at the base of the udder. The gland cister is poorly developed in the buffaloes because there is not accumulation of milk before milking in the gland cistern of buffaloes (Aliev, 1964). A series of branches of mammary ducts emerge from the gland cistern and ramify through sub-branches into the alveolar tissue and at the end forming terminal ductules for draining milk from the each avelous.

Development of Mammary Gland

The milk production in animals in mainly influenced by the quantity of milk synthesizing cells, the alveoli. The proportion of alveolar tissue is much higher than the connective tissue and other non-glandular tissues in the high milk producing buffaloes (Nosier, 1972).

(a) Prenatal development of mammary gland

The cellular differentiation of mammary tissue takes place in early embryonic life of 3 to 5 weeks of post-conception form the dermal cells in the inguinal region. The aggregation of mammary cells takes place duing the foetal development forming four distinct mammary buds, two in series on either side of the median line. The development of non-glandular tissues, viz., connective tissues and fat pad is almost complete at the time of birth and glandular part is rudimentary.

(b) Post natal development upto puberty

At birth although he formation of gland and teat cisterns are complete, the mammary duct system is stills short and limited to the region of the gland cistern. The growth of udder is slow inearly post-natal life upto 6-7 weeks and then increase steadily to a much faster rate than the body growth. In Egyptian buffalo heifers significant development tin the length and diameter of teats and the circumference of udder has been observed between 45 to 900 days of age, when the mammary glands reached functional stage (Nosier *et al.*, 1973). About 2-3 months before the onset of first oestrus a rapid proliferation of mammary parenchyma occurs. Cyclic changes exhibited by the accumulation of secretion in the lumina of smaller mammary ducts occur during the oestrus cycle and some regression is observed in latter in the oestrus cycle.

(c) Mammary growth during pregnancy

In the early phase of pregnancy more proliferation of mammary ducts occurs in the young heifers. The formation of interlobular ducts takes place and alveoli grow to replace the adipose tissue in the udder. The growth of grandular parenchyma is rapid throught ghe gestation period but the heifers it becomes econspicuous usually after 3-5 months of pregnancy. The size alveoli increases significantly during the terminal phase o pregnancy when udder becomes distended, smooth and bright in appearance.

(d) Mammary growth during lactation period

The multiplication of the cells of the mammary glands continues in the early phase of lactation, probably upto peak of lactation. Therefore, the alveoli are densely packed in the udder. During the declining phase of lactation the degeneration of glandular cells exceeds the formation of newer cells. The multiplication of mammary cells is maintained at a steady rate for longer duration in high milk producing buffaloes with longer lactation period.

(e) Mammary growth during dry period

Wide variations occur in the mammary gland of buffaloes during the dry period because it varies fromk less than 40 days to more than a year or so. Under normal breeding the buffaloes should be given a minimum 60 days of lactational rest otherwise milk production will be adversely affected in the following lactation. Partial to complete involution of udder occurs during the dry period depending on the length of dry period. Involution of udder is incomplete in females which conceive during the lactation period because the growth of mammary glands is stimulated by the hormones produced during the pregnancy.

Hormonal regulation of the development of mammary glands

Almost all the hormones required for the control of normal production also play significant role in the growth of mammary glands. This is evident from the fact that larger growth of mammary glands takes place during the puberty, pregnancy and a short period after the calveing. The hormones involved in mammary development are produced by anterior pituitary gland, ovaries, adrenal and thyroid glands and placenta.

i) **Anterior pituitary (hypophysis):** The growth hormone and prolactin stimulate the growth of mammary tissues and also had synergistic effect on the udder development stimulation of ovarian hormones, oestrogen and progesterone.

ii) **Ovaries:** Ovarian hormones, oestrogen and progesterone regulate the development of mammary glands during, puberty and pregnancy. The oestrogen stimulates the growth of mammary duct system whereas its combination with progesterone is required for the development of glandular parenchyma of the udder.

iii) **Adrenal and thyroid:** The stimulatory effect of the administration of adrenal steroids and thyroxine is perhaps related with their general stimulatory effect on metabolic activities in the body. The effect of these hormones on mammary growth is probably secondary.

iv) **Placental hormones:** Oestrogen and lactogen are the important hormones of placenta and they impart synergistic effect on the mammary growth alongwith hormones anterior pituitary gland and ovaries.

Udder Conformation

The shape and size of udder influence the lactational characteristics like milk ejection, milking time, rate of milk flow and also the milk yield (Polikhronov and Tosev, 1970; Nosier, 1972; Saxena and Prabhu, 1972; Sidhu and Pal, 1978; Turabov, 1982).

Shape of udder

The shape of buffalo udder has been distinguished in 3 to 5 types on basis of their appearance in the lactation females.

Three types of commonly described udder are bowl or trough shaped, round or globular shaped and goat type (Saxena and Prabhu, 1972; Saxena, 1973; Turabov and Abuliaev, 1979; Turabov, 1982). Pendulous type udder (Singh and Bhatnagar, 1977) and sub-grouping or round udders into bath-shaped and narrow-round shaped and primitive type adders (Saakoava, 1979) have been also identified in small herds of Indian and Caucasian buffaloes. Bowl shaped udders are prevalent and found in 70-75 percent Indian dairy buffaloes followed by round shaped in 14-18 percent and goat type in 8-12 percent animals of the organized herds. Round shaped udders are more in Caucasian buffaloes followed by bowl shaped and goat type.

Size of udder

The length, width and depth of udder and milk yield continue to increase upto third and fourth lactation after that there is gradual decrease in milk yield without any significant change in the size of udder (Saxena, 1973; Hafez and Naidu, 1981). Udder size is also significantly affected by stage of lactation and the number of lactation (Sindhu and Pal, 1978). The size of developed udder of Murrah type, Egyptian and Caucasian buffaloes is given in Table 3.1.

Table 3.1.

Udder traits (cm)	Murrah type (Saxena, 1973)	Caucasian (Saakova, 1979)	Egyptian (Alim, 1983)
Circumference	-	85.5±0.30	86.61±0.53
Length	54.81	32.46±0.74	-
Width	49.6	23.68±0.32	-
Depth	15.29	13.05±0.30	-
(i) Fore udder	-	-	15.91±0.10
(ii) Rear udder	-	-	14.41±0.09
Udder Score	-	-	1330.67±14.09

The size of udder decreases significantly after milking (Alim,1983).The multiplication fo alveolar cells of mammary gland is very rapid in the early lactation period and a gradual increase in udder size associated with the corresponding increase in milk yield is observed upto the peak yield after that gradual involution of udder and decline in milk yield takes place.

A little difference has been recorded in the udder shape of Murrah type buffaloes at the Military Dairy Farms in India and bowl shaped udder has been preferred. Almost linear increase in udder size and milk yield has been observed upto fourth lactation without a significant difference between the fourth and fifth lactation of the murrah type buffaloes at the organized dairy farms of India (Saxena, 1973). The length and width of udder shoed a declining trend in the fifth lactation but depth continues to increase (Table. 3.2).

Table 3.2. Effect of lactation number on udder size and test milk yield in Murrah buffaloes.

Traits	Lactation number				
	1	2	3	4	5
	Jabalpur Farm				
Udder Traits (cm)					
Length	49.30	53.22	55.25	58.00	58.09
Depth	44.64	48.88	50.66	52.46	51.04
Width	13.18	144.67	15.39	16.09	16.22
Milk yield (kg)	5.06	6.22	6.41	6.73	6.86
	Meerut Farm				
Udder Traits (cm)					
Length	51.00	55.15	56.84	60.67	58.51
Depth	49.23	50.36	53.24	57.01	53.61
Width	12.64	13.83	14.35	15.23	15.52
Milk yield (kg)	6.65	7.17	7.46	8.40	8.47

Some what similar trend has been reported in Egyptian buffaloes. Significant fall in udder circumference and udder score has been observed during the different stages of lactation being highest during the first two months of lactation period (Table. 3.3) in the Egyptian buffaloes (1983).

Table 3.3. Effect of lactation number and stage of lactation on udder size of Egyptian buffaloes.

Traits	Udder measurements (cm)			
	Front depth	Rear depth	Circum ference	Udder score
Number of lactation				
First	14.26	12.53	73.74	1004.02
Second to fourth	17.34	15.63	97.75	1613.43
Stage of lactation (month)				
First and second	16.17	14.63	98.09	1537.15
Third and fourth	15.75	14.10	88.85	1335.71
Over fifth	15.89	14.05	79.96	1229.19

Topography of udder

The udder of buffalo is situated in the inguinal region. The dairy type riverine buffaloes well developed udder is spread from just behind the ambicus to high upto third beneath the lower vulvar commisure and teats hand almost vertical in line with the ground surface. In Swamp buffaloes small size udder is placed posteriorly between the hind limbs and provide convenient disposition for the suckling of calves from the rear side through the space between the hind limbs. Rear suckling is quite common in the Swamp buffaloes. In Murrah type buffaloes distance from ventral end of vulva to rear attachment of udder to rear teat is 31.24 and 4.80 cm, from front attachmentof udder is 12.36±2.72 cm, from front attachment to fore teat is 11.21±2063 cm, udder length is 53.47±6.66 cm and the distance from ground to udder is 59.00±5.45 cm in a herd of organized farm (Mangurkar and Desai, 1981). The length of udder increases and the distance from ground decreases in the subsequent lactation. Changes in other measurements may be inconsistent (Table. 3.4).

Table 3.4. Effect of lactation number and stage of lactation on udder size of Egyptian buffaloes.

Udder measurements (cm)	Lactation Number					
	1	2	3	4	5	6
Distance from ventral end of vulva to rear attachment	12.36	11.84	12.23	12.03	11.75	12.80
Distance from rear attachmen of udder to rear teats	27.31	29.24	30.33	31.92	33.26	33.28
Distance from front attachment of udder to fore teats	9.86	10.74	11.31	10.94	11.99	12.34
Udder length Distance from ground to lowest end of teat	47.15	50.90	52.23	53.71	56.85	57.86
Udder length Distance from ground to lowest end of teat	61.41	59.04	58.31	57.82	55.49	56.71

Teats

The teat is a tubular terminal continuation of the each quarter of the udder and its main function is the drainage of milk from the mammary gland at the time of suckling and milking. The flow of milk is controlled by the strong sphincter muscles around the streak canal.

The teat is made of external epidermis, which is thicker towards the orifice, middle layer of corium of dense connective tissues with numerous blood capillaries and lymphatic ramification and the inner subcutaneous layer is composed of white fibrous tissue, elastic fibres and a few bundles of smooth muscle fibres. The teat skin is free from hair follicles and sweat and sebaceous glands. The teat cistern starts narrow from the streak canal and widens upwards to continue as the poorly developed udder cistern. The tunica epithelialis of teat canal is formed of a single layer of cuboidal cells resting on a basement membrane. Numerous folds project from the mucosa (Fahmy *et al.,*., 1969).

(a) Shape of teats

Three types of normal teats are found in dairy buffaloes, viz., cylindrical, conical and funnel shaped. The first two types are more common and found in 70-80 percent of buffaloes (Bhosrekar and Nagpaul, 1971, Saxena and Prabhu, 1972; Singh and Bhatnagar, 1977), Variation in teat shape of fore and rear quarters of the same buffalo is frequently observed.

(b) Size of teats

Moderate size evenly placed teats provide convenient disposition both for hand milking and the machine milking. The rear teats are usually longer and voluminous than the fore teats. Age, number of lactation and the stage of lactation significalty effect the size of teats (nosier *et al.,*., 1973; Sidhu and Pal, 1978; Saa kova, 1979; Alim, 1983). The mean length and diameter of teats in a herd of Caucasian buffalo has been recorded to be 6.64 cm and 1.60 cm for the fore teats and 8.03 and 1.93 cm for the rear teats, respectively (Saakova, 1979) and these measurement of corresponding teats in Murrah buffaloes are 7.50±0.72 and 2.65±0.04 cm and 8.50±0.13 and 2.83±0.04cm (Sidhu and Pal, 1980), Milking has significant effect on the size of teats (Table 3.5), Usually length increases and diameter decreases after the milking of buffaloes, which return to original position before the next milking time (Aliev *et al.,* 1965; Alim, 1983). A large variation in the in the teat size ranging from 1.1 to 3.7 cm in diameter and 2.7 to 9.6 cm in length has been reported. A teat length of less than 6.64 cm and diameter below 1.60 cm are generally not suitable for machine milking (Gotsiridze and Saakova, 1980).

Table 3.5. Change in size of teats after milking

Milking Effect	Teat length (cm)		Teat circumference (cm)	
	Fore	Rear	Fore	Rear
Left size				
Before Milking	7.86±0.04	8.87±0.06	3.30±0.02	3.34±0.02
After Milking	8.58±0.03	9.23±0.04	2.83±0.02	2.90±0.02
Right side				
Before Milking	8.02±0.046	9.12±0.05	3.14±0.02	3.49±0.02
After Milking	8.78±0.03	9.58±0.04	2.90±0.02	3.09±0.02

(c) Placement of teats

Similar to length and diameter there is also large variation in the placement of teats. Even size squarely placed teats are convenient for milking. The distance between the four teats is larger when the udder is distended before the milking, which comes closer after the milking due to sunkening of the udder (Table 3.6). The distance between front teats and between eh rear teats is often adequate but often less between the side teats for efficient milking (Alim, 1983). Average distance between the fore teats and between the fore teats and between the fore and reat teats in a herd of Murrah buffaloes has been recorded to be 13.44±0.14 cm and 8.94±0.13 cm, respective (Sidhu and Pal, 1980).

Table 3.6. Distance between the teats of Egyptian buffalo before and after milking.

Particulars	Distance between teats (cm)
Between force teats	
Before milking	13.71±0.077
After milking	11.39±0.067
Between rear teats	
Before milking	9.23±0.061
After milking	7.95±0.053
Between force teats	
Before milking	7.41±0.049
After milking	6.49±0.044
Between force teats	
Before milking	7.42±0.066
After milking	6.46±0.042

Anomalies of Udder and Teats

Several anomalies of udder and teats have been reported in buffaloes.

(a) Udder anomalies

An unique case of hypoplasis of udder in twin buffalo heifers born in Sumartra presented satisfactory evidence of mirror imaging requirement of the monozygous twins. One heifer lacked a teat on right fore quarter and the other on left forequarter and both had unilateral hppoplasia of the udder on different sides (fischer, 1956). In a mixed herd of 66 Murrah, 380 Murrah grades and 184 mondescript female buffaloes, the incidence of udder anomalies was about 4.91 percent, which included about 1.58, 1.75 and 158 percent incidence of hyposlas, cloven udders, and hyper and hypo mastia, respectively (Rao and Murthy, 1984).The prevalence of mammary gland anomalies was much higher in Murrah buffaloes.

(b) Teat anomalies

The various teat anomalies encountered in buffaloes are the fused teats, pouched teats, blind teats and supernumerary teats. The fusion of fore and rear teats of left side has been observed in Murrah buffalo. In another animal there were five functional teats (Fischer, 1962). An incidence of 4.91 percent fused teats, 1.93 percent pouched teats and 2.28 percent supernumerary teats has been reported in a mixed herd of 630 female buffaloes of Murrah, braded Murrah and nondescript breeds (Rao and Murthy, 1984). A large variation ranging from 2.28 to 37.9 percent in the occurrence of supernumetary teats has been reported in the Indian dairy buffaloes (Dwivedi and Prabhu, 1970; Ludri and Sarma, 1981; Verma *et al.*, 1984). The incidence of supernumerary teats in hders of Murrah, Mehsana, Jaffarabadi, crossbred and graded buffaloes has been found to e about 2.60, 1.34, 2.33, 8. 65 and 2.67 percent, respectively, which was lowest in Mehsana breed. The occurrence at intercalary position (between the normal teats) is more than the caudal and renal position. About 1.8 percent supernumerary teats were functional. The incidence of single supernumerary teats was about 2.25 percent, where as two supernumerary teats were found only in about 0.34 percent animals (Dwivedi and prabhu, 1970). Author has recorded river buffaloes having only two and three teats.

Lactation

The process of milk secretion from the mammary gland is known as lactation. The milk constituents are partly contributed by the blood and largely produced in the alveoli of the mammary glands. There is no significant difference in the osmotic pressure of milk and blood, but there is significant difference in their composition. The milk of buffalo is white in colour whereas normal colour of blood is bright red. The concentration of protein in milk is lower thatn the blood but those of sugar, fat, calcium, phosphorus and potassium is much higher. Sodium and chloride contents are also les in milk which increases considerably durig the declining phase of lactation. The milk protein is mostly casein with small amounts of albumin and globulins. The latter are much more in the first milk, colostrums. On the other hand albumins and globulins are the main proteins of blood. The milk fat is largely triglycerides and principal components of blood lipids are cholesterol and phospholipids.

Under normal conditions lactation in buffaloes starts immediately after the parturition when stimulated by the suckling of calf. The first milk is colostrums, which contains very high concentration of fat, proteins, immunoglobulins and ash and low level of lactose in comparison to normal milk. In dairy buffaloes the milk secretion increases steadily to attain peak yield at 3-10 weeks of lactation period in different breeds of buffaloes (Maymone, 1945; Malosini, 1967; Kumar and Bhat, 1969; Chowdhary and Chaudhary, 1981).

The following terminologies are commonly used for describing the lactation (i) lactation or galactophoesis is the complete process of secretion and removal of milk from the udder, (ii) initiation of lactation or milk secretion is referred to the intracellular synthesis of milk and its subsequent drainage from the cytoplasma into the lumen of alveoli, (iii) milk ejection or let down of milk is the active process of milk removal from the udder due to the contraction of myoepithelial cells surrounding the alveoli. This function is initiated by the action of oxytocin either liberated intrinsic from the posterior pituitary gland or injected pharmaceutical preparation, and (iv) milk removal involves both active action of oxytocin and passive removal by suckling of calf or milk.

Hormonal control of lactation

Although several hormones are involved in the initiation and maintenance of milk secretion, the precise mechanism of lactation is not yet known. The milk production capacity of buffaloes depends on the ratio of glandular and non-glandular tissues in the mammary gland, which is wider in heavy yields (Nosier, 1972). The estrogen stimulates the growth of mammary duct system and in combination with progresterone the growth of labuloalveolar tissue (Shalash et l., 1961; Ferrara *et al.,*. 1966, Sud and Singh, 1974). For the complete development of the mammary gland pituitary hormones are also necessary alongwith the oestrogen and progesterone. The prolactin and adenocorticotropic hormone (ACTH) and important for the initiation and maintenance of lactation. ACTH maintains the required levels of various milk precursors in the blood. Thyroxine has temporary effect on increasing the production of milk but it is not essential for the galactopoieses (Asker *et al.,*., 1954; Allev, 1962). The pituitary hormone, oxygen is responsible for the milk ejection nand frequently used for the let down of milk in the difficult animals (Chandiramani *et al.,*., 1966; Jadhav and Kambata, 1967; Hanna *et al.,*., 1979). The oxytocin stimulates the contraction of the myoephithelial cells around the alveoli and along the mammary ducts and milk secretion starts.

Initiation of lactation

At the time of parturition the level of prolaction and ACTH increases and that of oestrogen and progesterone decreases. This marked change in the level of different hormones is responsible for the initiation of lactation.

Maintenance of lactation

The maintenance of lactation in buffaloes is influenced by the hormones and the husbandry practices like optimum balanced feeding, water supply and bath or wallowing, maintenance of health and regularity in milk. In buffaloes gentle massage with warm water in weaned buffaloes and suckling stimulates the release of hormones. Unlike cows there is no accumulation of milk in the cistern and thus the suppression of lactation due to high infra-mammary pressure is probably and important in buffaloes (Aliev, 1962). The ratio between secretory cells at the stage of formation, the actively functioning cells and the cells under the process of involution varies in different stages of lactation. The ratio of cells under involution increases in the declining phase of lactation period. Actively functional cells are maximum during the peak lactation. It is assumed that the individual groups of secretory cells at different stages of their development form qualitatively different secretory -motor complexes are functionally different from one another due to which milk of different fat percentage is obtained in the consecutive portions of a single yield (Table. 3.7).

Table: 3.7. Fat content in different portions of milk of a single miling at different stage of lactation.

Portions of milk	Fat content (%) at different months		
	1st month	4th months	7th months
1	6.01	9.97	9.10
2	5.19	9.20	10.00
3	4.77	7.13	12.40
4	4.95	7.90	14.61
5	6.35	9.50	-
6	7.72	11.20	-
7	10.76	-	-

Milk ejection or let down of milk

The mechanism of the transfer of milk from the functional alveoli into the mammary ducts and its subsequently flow from the mammary gland through the orifice of teats is known as milk ejection or let down or milk. The process is initiated by a stimulus for releasing the oxytocin hormone from the posterior lobe of the prituitary gland. The oxytocin is quickly transported in blood to the mammary tissue, where it produces contraction of the myoepithelial eels surrounding the alveoli. The milk is expelled from the alveoli into the duct system to finally enter the cisterns of the udder and teats. This causes sudden rise of internal pressure in the cistern. At this stage milk is easily removed by the suckling of calf or milking. The complete process is governed by afferent motor nerve and the hormone, oxytocin and this reflex action is known as neuron-hormonal or neuron-endocrine reflex.

In dairy buffaloes, this reflex becomes conditional and can be stimulated by the specific sounds of ratling milk pails, the application of teat cup in machine milking, the washing of udder, movement to milking byre, massage by the milker and suckling of calf.

Significant change in surrounding area distribing the animal may greatly influence the let down of milk e.g. in case of suckling when the calf is tied away from the normal practice of keeping near the dam, the animal gets agitated and milk let down is incomplete and secretion of fat in different portions of milk is irregular (Alive, 1971). Oxytocin is effective for a very short duration of 3-10 minutes (Shafie *et al.*, 1971; Gupta *et al.*, 1974; Dass *et al.*, 1976; Alim, 1983; Roay and Nagpaul, 1984).

Induced lactation

Infertility and sub-fertility are the serious reproductive disorders of buffaloes. Most of these animals are either culled in active production life for slaughter or maintained barren for several years without any return. Establishment of active lactation in such buffaloes can be helpful in obtaining the large amount of milk going waste in these animals. Various degrees of udder growth and lactation have been achieved by hormonal treatments in barran buffaloes. Adminsitration of oestrogen and progesterone stimulated the growth of udder and teats, initiated milk production and maintained lactation for different durations (Shalash *et al.,.,* 1961). Biopsy of udder showed different stages of alveolar growth i.e. resting parenchyma tissue, various degree of growth in parenchyma and milking lobules and acini (D' Angelo and DeFranciscis, 1966). The response of hormonal induction of lactation has been poor in young buffalo heifers of 15-18 monghs of age (Shyalash *et al.*, 1966a, b) but in adult infertile heifers of 4-6 years and buffaloes of 6-13 years encouraging results have been obtained (Sud, 1979; Rao *et al.*, 1982; Atheya and Sud, 1985). Gross composition of milk was comparable in both types of buffaloes (Table 3.8).

Table 3.8. Chemical composition of milk from normal and induced lactation buffaloes.

Milk constituents (%)	Young heifers Induced milk		Adult buffaloes Normal	Induced	Normal
	1st milk	Last milk	milk	milk	milk
Milk fat	5.81	6.809	7.48	8.71	6.42
Protein	20.05	4.60	3.95	4.13	4.24
Lactose	0.65	3.42	4.90	4.40	4.53
Ash	3.18	0.85	0.80	0.73	0.73
Casein	7.73	3.68	3.16	-	-
Solid not fat	23.88	8.87	9.65	8.53	8.30

For the artificial induction of lactation in barren buffaloes hormones are administered by sub-cutaneous injection , as sub-cutaneous implant in the neck region followed by sub-cutaneous injection after 6 weeks or alongwith udder induction of diethylstillboesterol dipropionate. So afar these treatments are in the experimental stage and have not been accepted for routine use.

Hormonal stimulation of lactation

Thyroxing and various iodinated proteins like thyroidin and thyroprotein have shown stimulatory effect on the lactation in buffaloes (Asker *et al.,.,* 1954; Moqsood, 1956; Aliev, 1962). An increase upto 19 percent in milk yield and 42 percent in milk fat may occur due to the administration of thyroine. The administration of thyroxine in the beginning of lactation mainly stimulates the secretion of milk, at the peak of lactation the secretion of both milk and milk fat and during the declining phase of lactation it limits the drop in milk yield and increases the fat percentage in the milk. It has complicated effect on the secretion of milk production, which is primarily affected by the stage of lactation. In the beginning of lactation, which is primarily affected by the stage of lactation. In the beginning of lactation usually there is no change in the protein percentage of milk but total production is high due to increase in milk yield. At the peak of lactation it increases protein percentage as well as yield. In the declining phase of lactation and small doses of thyro-active substances do not have significant effect but the administration of larger doses increases protein content (Aliev, 1971). The administration of larger doses increases protein content (Aliev, 1971). The administration of thyroprotein should be accompanied by the feeding of the higher level of energy. The use of thyroactive substance for increasing the milk production is not practiced due to inconsistent effect in the subsequent lactation.

Adverse effect of hypothyroidism produced by the feeding of the methylthiouracil on lactation and accelerated involution of the secretory cells of the mammary gland has been observed, it causes sudden drop in milk yield but increase in the milk fat percentage (Aliev, 1971).

Biosyntheis of Milk

The milk is composed of water, milk fat, proteins lactose, minerals and vitamins. Some leucocytes, shaded mammary cells and enzymes are also present. The biosynthesis of milk depends on the extraction of nutrients from the blood by the mammary cells, conversion of blood nutrients into the milk constituents and the discharge of milk from the alveoli into the alveolar lumen.

Secretory cells of the mammary gland

Each functional state of mammary gland is characterized by the development pattern of the secretory cells, which are at different stages of differentiation. The ratio between the secretory cells and non-secretory tissue is very wide in the nonlactating growing heifers upto about 31 months of age, which becomes narrower due to faster proliferatio of the glandular tissue during the puberty (Table. 3.9). The right half of udder contains more glandular tissue than the left half, which is either due to the difference in blood supply to the two sides of the udder or it may be the characterstics of buffaloes (El-Sheikh and Sultan, 1077). The ratio between the glandular and non-glandular tissues changes significantly.int eh functional udder due to many fold quantitative and qualitative increase in the glandular tissue. The proportion of glandular tissue is much higher in the high milk yielding buffaloes than the low yielding buffaloes (Nosier, 1972). It is assumed that the individual group of secretory cells at different stages of their development constitutes qualitatively different secretory-motor complexes of the udder. These complexes are distinguished form one another on the basis of their synthesis ability of different milk components, the nature of secretory processes and the ability to discharge the synthesized milk (Olenov, 1954).

Table 3.9. Mean area (cm2) of secretory (S) and non-secretory (NS) tissues of development mammary gland at different ages in buffalo heifers.

Parts of udder	Age of heifers in months				
	13	18	24	31	37
Left fore					
S	14.5	14.9	14.9	18.5	17.6
NS	228.3	259.3	239.8	249.3	226.3
NS-S	15.74	17.40	16.09	13.48	12.86
Right fore					
S	15.0	20.6	16.3	18.5	23.7
NS	233.5	247.7	242.0	231.7	253.6
NS-S	15.57	12.02	14.85	12.52	10.70

Left rear					
S	16.4	16.5	20.6	15.8	22.3
NS	270.4	252.9	254.0	230.2	192.6
NS-S	16.49	15.33	12.70	14.67	8.64
Right rear					
S	21.2	25.6	22.6	20.6	21.5
NS	226.5	247.3	243.7	248.1	217.6
NS-S	10.68	9.66	10.78	12.04	10.12
Whole udder					
S	16.8	19.4	18.7	18.4	21.3
NS	236.7	251.6	244.9	239.8	222.5
NS-S	14.09	12.97	13.10	13.03	10.45

The mammary cell is highly active during the lactation with very high rate of metabolism for the synthesis of the various milk constituents (Patton, 1969). Functional mammary cells obtain large quantity of milk precursors like glucose, acetate, amino acids and minerals from the blood and during the active lactation phase high milk yield animals may loose body tissue to meet the heavy nutrients requirement of the mammary gland.

Structure of secretory cell of mammary gland

The epithelial cells in alveoli are the secretory cells. A functional secretory cell is situated on the basement membrane of outer connective tissue, blood capillaries and the inner layer of myoepithelial cells. Each cell is enveloped in a plasma membrane in addition to a well defined nucleus. The various cytoplamic inclusions are the mitochondria, Golgi apparatus, endoplasmic reticulum, lysosome, fat droplets and protein micelles.

Nucleus: Nucleus of mammary cells is responsible for the transmission of inherent lactation characteristics in the genes for the synthesis of milk proteins and certain enzymes required for the catalysis of many biochemical reactions in the secretory cell. The deoxyribonucleic acid (DNA) in the chromosome of nucleus possesses the genetic information, which is passed on to ribonucleic acid (RNA). The RNA carries the information to endoplasmic reticulum through the fine pores in the nuclear membrane.

Endoplasmic reticulum: The specialized organelle found int eh basal part of cytoplasm in the secretory cell is made of a canal system. The RNA moves the specific message from the nucleus to the endoplasmic reticulum and transmits information for the linkage of the different amino acids for the synthesis of milk proteins and the enzymes in the mammary cell. The surface of some of the canals of proteins and the enzymes in the mammary cell. The surface of some of the canals of the endoplasmic reticulum is lodged with the RNA protein combination known as ribosomes. The synthesis of milk proteins from the linage between peptide bonds of amino acids in different sequence occurs on the ribosomes.

Golgi apparatus: The packaging of proteins like combination of calcium and phosphorus with the casein micelles takes place in the Golgi apparatus. After synthesis milk protein emerges out of the Golgi apparatus in small vacuoles which fuse with the plasma membrane. Lactose synthesis also takes place in the Golgi apparatus.

Mitochondria: Several mitochondria are present in the active secretory cells of mammary gland. These organelle generate energy for the synthesis of milk proteins and fats in the cell.

Lysosomes: These are membranes bound particles and the integrity of lysosomal membranes is maintained by the hormones. The leakage of degradative lysosomal engymes into the cytoplasm activates the digestion and removal of the cell from the body. The lysosomes are more active during the involution of glandular tissue of the mammary gland, which occurs with the end of lactation period and in early dry period.

Cellular membranes: Each Secretary cell of the mammary gland is enveloped in the plasma membrane. The various organelles in the cytoplasm are enclosed in separate membranes, which are very specific for the passage of chemicals into various compartments of the cell. Although milk is isotonic with the blood but there is large difference in the normal constituents of both the fluids. Milk contains many times higher fat, sugar, calcium, phosphorus and potassium and lower amount of sodium and protein than the blood of the same animal.

Cytoplasm: The larger portion of mammary cell is constituted of cytoplasm. Cytoplasm contains soluble and colloidal form of many nutrients, enzymes and other cytoplasmic inclusions.

Milk proteins: The primary proteins of milk are caseins, lactabumin and lactoglobulins which are synthesized in the mammary cells from the free amino acids received from the blood. The other group of proteins comprising of immune globulins and milk serum albumin are also received from the blood and remain unchanges in the milk.

Lactose: The main sugar of milk is a disaccharide, factose, which is made of one molecule each of glucose and galactose. The only precursor of lactose received from the blood in the mammary cell is glucose. Two molecules of glucose are required for the formation of one molecule of lactose. For this purpose, one molecule of glucose is first converted into galactose, which combines with a molecule of glucose. The reaction is catalyzed by an enzyme, lactose synthesis and one unit of this enzyme is alpha factalbumin.

Milk Fat: The milk fat is mostly mixed triglyceriods containing high proportion of short chain fatty acids. Milk fat also contains larger proportion of saturated fatty acids. The short chain fatty acids are synthesized to the secretory cells of mammary gland from the volatile fatty acids, acetic acid and butyric acid produced during the microbial fermatation fo the dietary carbohydrates in the rumino-reticulum and absorbed in the body pool. Most of the long chain fatty acids of milk fat are contributed diretly by the feed lipids. Fatty acids of plant origin are almost unsaturated long chain fatty acids, which undergo various degree of saturation in the rumen. These saturated long chain fatty acids are absorbed from the intestine into lymphatic system. In the lymph lacteals fatty acids bind with a protein and then transmitted to the blood stream and carried to mammary gland. The secretory cells of mammary gland absorb these fatty acids from the blood, which ultimately form the part of milk fat.

Vitamins and minerals: The entire quantity of vitamins and minerals in the secretory cell of mammary gland are obtained from the blood through the selective permeability and they are not synthesized in the mammary parenchyma.

Water in milk: Water in milk is derived from two sources i.e. (a) from blood and (b) from the high potassium intracellular fluid of the alveolar cells. The synthesis of lactose, fat and protein in the secretory cell stimulates the flow of water fro the blood for the maintenance of osmotic equilibrium between the milk and blood. Buffalo milk contains about 82 percent water.

Milking of Buffalo

System of milking: Hand milking is extensively followed for the milking of buffaloes, but on some organized farms machine milking is also practiced. Dairy buffaloes are normally milk two times daily at an interval of about 12 hours, whereas in low milk yielding swamp buffaloes once dairy milking is usually followed.

Hand milking: Usually two methods of hand milking i.e. full hand milking and stripping are practiced. The former is used for the milking of well developed large teats and latter for the small size teats. A third method of hand milking known as fisting or knuckling is rarely used for milking of hard teats. This method is injuries to teats and may be predisposing cause of infection leading to mastitis.

Full hand milking: The teat is held with the thumb and the first finger in the fist and milk is squeezed out applying adequate pressure by the palm and fingers. The process is repeated at a fast rate in quick succession. The method is rarely used for the milking of buffaloes because teats of buffaloes are sufficiently long and voluminous for the full hand milking.

Stripping: In this method ....

Precautions observed at milking: The following precautions need to be observed at the time milking:

a) Milking paid and byre should be clean and free from flies and offensive odours.

b) Milker should wash hands and rinse in a solution fo potassium permanganate.

c) Udder should be washed and wiped dry with a clean cloth before milking.

d) Fist milk streams should be drawn on stip cup for clinical examinations.

e) Knuckling or fisting of udder should not be permitted.

f) Strangers should not be allowed.

g) Animals should be handled gently and should not be annoyed.

Milking duration: The total time of milking includes the pre-milking stimulation or time for the let down of milk and the milking duration.

i) **Milk let down time:** It ranges from 30 seconds to 300 seconds in different buffaloes, and it is influenced by several factors (Dass *et al.*, 1976; Gangwar *et al.*, 1980. Alim *et al.*, 1982; Goy and Nagpaul, 1984. Some factors affecting the pre-milking stimulation or let down time are as follows:

a) **Normal milking schedule:** Twice a day milking at a regular interval of about 12 hours is the normal milking practice in buffaloes. Milk let down time in Murrah buffaloes is 0.5 – 4.0 minutes (Gupta *et al.*, 1974; Dass *et al.*, 1974: Ludri, 1980; Roy and Nagpaul, 1984) and in Egyptian buffaloes 2.72±0.89 minutes at the morning milk and 2.82±0.92 minutes at the evening milking when udder is massaged with a warm cloth squeezed in water at 104-105°F (Alim *et al.*, 1982).

b) **Frequency of milking:** Milk let down time in Murrah buffaloes increased significantly from 113±7.36 seconds in case of two time daily milking to 137±10.04 seconds on the three times daily milk at equal interval between the milking (Dass *et al.*, 1976).

c) **Stage of lactation:** The let down time of milk slightly decreased during the third month of lactation period and thereafter increased significantly. It varies widely between the animals and has been found to be 50-256 (Av. 123) seconds during 31-60 days of lactation perod, 32-10 (Av. 120) second beteen 61.90 days and 32-319 (Av. 146) seconds between 91-120 days and 50-300 (Av. 146) seconds between 121-150 days of lactation period in Murrah buffaloes maintained under the standard management practices of an organized farm (Ludri, 1980).

d) **Effect of weaning:** Early weaning of buffaloes increases the milk let down time and it has been observed to be 133-172.5 seconds in early weaned, 86.4-100 seconds in late weaned and 97.5-104 seconds in the unweaned Murrah buffaloes (Gupta *et al.*, 1974).

e) **Effect of envorinmental cooling and season:** The environmental cooling arrangements like shower bath and wallowing during the dry-hot and humid-hot season significantly increased the milk let down time. The mean milk let down time has been found to be 3.105, 3.683 and 4.154

minutes in buffaloes without bath, given shower bath and wallowing, respectively during the dry season and the corresponding figures for humid season are 3.089, 3.501 and 3680 minutes (Gangwar *et al.,* 1980).

f) **Effect of udder massage:** Massage of udder before milking with a cloth squeezed in warm water at 1.04-105°F increases the pre-milking stimulation time in Egyptain buffaloes. Mean let down time is about 4.39±1.30 minutes on dry hand massage and 5.31±1.51 minutes on wet massage with warm cloth for twice dairy milking (Alim *et al.,* 1982).

g) **Effect of temperament:** Milk let down time in docile buffaloes is about 120.83 seconds which increases significantly to 295.32 seconds in nervous buffaloes producing 9.81 and 7.89 kg milk daily (Roy and Nagpaul, 1984a).

ii) **Milking duration:** Milking duration varies from 5-13 minutes in different types of buffaloes (Shafle *et al.,* 1971; Turabov and Abullave, 1979; Gangwar *et al.,* 1980; Tsankova and Tosev, 1980, Alim *et al.,* 1982; Roay and Nagpaul, 1984b). On machine milking also almost equal time is required (Aliev *et al.,* 1071; Gotsiridze and Saakova, 1980). The time required for the milking of buffaloes is influenced by the following factors:

a) **Time of milking:** Milking duration is usually longer in morning than in the evening which is mainly due to more milk production in the morning milking (Shafie *et al.,* 1971; Alim *et al.,* 1977; 1982).

b) **Effect of lactation number:** The duration of milking increases significantly upto the third lactation. The average machine milking time has been found to be 6.39, 8.47 and 10.26 minutes at the milking rate of 0.74, 0.77 and 0.99 kg per minute in the first, second and third lactations, respectively (Gotsiridze and Saakova, 1980). In a hand milked herd of Causcasian buffaloes average milking time in the first, second and third lactation at the flow rate of 0.56, 0.61 and 0.67 kg per minute has been found to e 7.08, 8.30 and 9.46 minutes, respectively (Turabov, 1982). Milk yield on the day was 4.13, 5.37 and 6.35 kg in the respective lactations.

c) **Effect of udder shape:** The shape of udder has marked effect on the milking duration. The bowl or cup shaped and round udders yield more milk than the goat type udder and require much less time for the complete milking (Saakova, 1979, Turabov and Abulaev, 1979; Turabov, 1982). Milking duration varies from 6.27±8.97 minutes for bowl shaped, 8.72±9.64 minutes for found and 8.19-13.67 minutes for goat type udders.

d) **Effect of udder quarters:** Milking of fore quarters of udder requires less time than the rar quarter, because fore quarter secrete abtou 30-42 percne tof Total milk production of the particular milking (Polikhronov and Tosev, 1970 and Tosev, 1980, Pandey *et al.,* 1981, Alim *et al.,* 1982.

e) **Effect of udder massage:** The wet massage of udder with a warm cloth squeezed in water at 104-105°F and dry massage took almost equal time of the milking (Alim *et al.,* 1977, 1982). Light massage of udder during milk markedly reduced the duration of milking. Massage of udder also affected the rate of milk flow and higher contribution of milk from the forequarters of bidder (Gostridze and kitoshvili, 1981).

f) **Effect of environment cooling:** The milking time of buffaloes is influenced by the cooling arrangements. Shower bath increases milking duration due to significant reduction in the flow rate of milk, whereas wallowing has little effect (Gangwar *et al.,* 1980).

g) **Effect of temperament:** Docile buffaloes require less time than the nervous buffaloes for the milking of the equal amount of milk, because the flow rate of milk in nervous buffaloes is usually low (Roy and Nagpaul, 1984; Gupta *et al.,* 1985).

Rate of Milking on Milk Flow Rate

The Flow rate of milk from the udder during the time of milking is an important factor in milking management. Large variation occurs in the milk flow rate, which is influenced by several factors. It varies from 0.21 -0-.99 kg per minute in different animals being highest in bowl and round udders and lowest in goat type udders (Ragab *et al.,* 1971; Alim *et al.,* 1977, 1987; Gangwar *et al.,* 1980; Gotsiridze and Kitoshvili, 1981; Turabov, 1982; Kapoor and Ludri, 1984; Roy and Nagpaul, 1984). The effect of various factors on the flow rate of milk is as follows:

Effect of the number of lactation: The flow rate of milk increases linear in the subsequent lactations. The flow rate may be different in the different herds of buffaloes depending upon the skill of the milker, type of animals and the system milking. Mean flow rate on machine milking in a herd of Caucasian buffaloes has been recorded to be 0.74, 0.77 and 0.99 kg per minute in the first, second and third lactation, respectively (Gotsiridze and Saakova, 1980). In the same order of lactation, the mean flow rate of milk in a hand milked herd was 0.56, 0.61 and 0.67 kg per minute (Turabov, 1982).

Effect of the shape of udder: The milking of bowl and round shaped udders is more easy and efficient both the hand milking as well as the machine milking (Turabov and Adbulacv, 1979, Turabov, 1982). The goat type udder is difficult to milk and has been unsuitable for the machine milking (Gostsiridze and Saakova, 1980).

Effect of the udder quarters: The milking rate is invariably higher for the rear quarters than the fore quarters probably due to the higher percentage of total milk yield in the near quarter (Alim *et al.,* 1982).

Effect of milking frequency: Twice daily milking at an interval of 12 hours is the common practice and milk flow rate is usually more at the time of morning milking than the afternoon milking (Alim *et al.,* 1982). On increasing milking frequency from the normal twice daily to trice daily at an interval of 8 hours about 15.5 percent decrease in milk flow rate occurred (Dass *et al.,* 1976). However, such trend could not be observed in another herd of Murrah buffaloes milked at 4, 8, 12 and 16 hours interval (Kapoor and Ludri, 1984).

Effect of udder massage: Premilking massage of udder significantly increases the flow rate of milk upto 25.7 percent and also the total yield of milk and the length of the lactation period (Gotsiridze and kitoshvili, 1981). The system of udder massage does not significantly influence the flow rate of milk from the udder (Alim *et al.,* 1977, 1982).

Effect of body cooling and season: A marginal increase in milk flow rate occurs in buffaloes allowed wallowing before the milking but shower baths adversely affect during the drya hot season. In humid season of tropical India wallowing increases the flow rate of milk (Soni, 1975).

Effect of temperament: Contrary to very high increase in let down time of milk in nervous and aggressive buffaloes, only little slower rate of milk flow rate occurs in comparison to docile buffaloes (Roy and Nagpaul, 1984; Gupta *et al.,* 1985).

Effect of milking machine: The type of milking machine significantly affects the milk flow rate and the machine with an arrangement of mechanical udder stimulation mechanism through gentle massage gives best results (Aliev *et al.,* 1971). The pulsation rates and the pressure in machine during the time of milking also influence the rate of milk. At the rate of 60 pulsation per minute at 40 cm Hg pressure the performance of 'Stimul' machine has been found to be superior (Aliev and Kuliev, 1965).

Residual Milk or complementary Milk

A small amount of milk remains in the udder after normal milking and it is known as residual or complementary milk. Since the cistern milk is almost negligible in buffaloes, very little amount of milk is left unstrapped in the udder (Aliev *et al.,* 1965). Residual milk may be obtained by the administration of 10 IU oxytocin injection, which is usually less thatn half litre (Aliev, 1966, Jadhav and Ekambata, 1967; Ludri, 1980). Residual milk contains very high percentage of milk fat. Administration of oxytocin by subcutaneous or inframuscular route has no significant effect on its letdown effect (Hanna *et al.,* 1979) and due to this reason oxytocin and posterior pituitary injections are indiscriminately used by the owners of private dairy buffaloes.

Involution or Regression of the Udder

In buffaloes regression of the glandular parenchyma is a slow and gradual process. Due to this character buffaloes have long lactation period ranging form 270-352 days in Murrah, about 350 days in Surti and 276 days in Bhdawari (Bhat, 1979). In Egyptain buffaloes lactation period ranges from 245-263 days in the different herds (Ragab, 1979) and in Swamp buffaloes of Thailand from 210-333 days (Chantalakahana, 1979). Still longer period sometimes as long as two year sis occasionally encountered in some buffaloes. The regression of mammary gland starts after the peak yiueld in declining phase of lactation period and it is enhanced by pregnancy, weaning of calf and irregular milking.

An Unusual Case of Spontaneous Lactation in a Virgin Buffalo

An unbred buffalo heifer developed functional udder without mating, calving or any other treatment at about three and half years of age and starled milk secretion. Teh heifer was milked for five years and yielded about 5-6 seers of normal milk equivalent to about 4.5-5.5 kg (Bali, 1962). Instance of milk production without breeding and also for 2-3 years after first calving are heard in the Indian villages, but mostly such information are unrecorded wheresay.

References

Aliev, M.G. 1962. Effect of thyroxine on the secretion of milk and butter fat. Doki, Akad. Nauk., Azerb., 18(6): 67-70.

Aliev, M.G. 1964. The physiology of lactation in buffaloes. Baku. Izdateijstvo Akad., Nauk., Azerb, 188 pp.

Aliev, M.G. 1971. Milk secretion in buffaloes. Dairy Sci. abst. 33:175-180.

Aliev, M.G. and Kuliev, K.M. 1965. Effect of different pulsation rates of the milking machine "Stimuli' on milk ejection in buffaloes. Trudy. Sekt., Fiziol., Kaku, 8: 55-66.

Aliev, M.G. Kuliev, K.M. and Mamedov, N.G. 1965a. External changes of the teat during the milking of buffaloes. Trudy Sekt., Fiziol., Baku, 8: 46-54.

Aliev, M.G., Kuliev, K.M. and Mamedov, N.G. 1965b. hand stripping after machine milking of buffaloes. Trudy Sekt. Fiziol., Baku, 8: 67-71.

Aliev, M.G., Kuliev, K.M. and Abbasov, S. 1971. Effedtiveness of mechanical stimulation in the milking of buffalo cow. Tekhnika sel'khoz., Mosk., 31(5): 28-30.

Alim, K.A. 1983. Repeatability of milking characteristics and udder triats in buffaloes. World Rev. Anim. Prod., 19(3): 13-18.

Alim, K.A., Barbari, A. and Badran, A. 1977. Management trials on milking technique and concentrate feeding with local cattle and buffalo. World Rev., Anim. Prod. 13(s): 27-32.

Alim, K.A.., Barbari, A. and Feel, F.M. 1982. Aspects of milking technique and productivity of udder quarters in buffalo. World Rev., Anim Prod., 18(1): 33-41.

Asker, A.A., Ragab, M.T. and Kamal, T.H. 196\54. The effect of feeding thyroprotein on the composition of milk of Egyptian buffaloes. Indian J. of Dairy Sci., 7: 36-39.

Atheya, U.K.J.a nd Sud, S.C. 1985. Hormonal induction of lactation of infertile aged buffaloes. Indian J. Anim. Sci. 55: 236-240.

Badawl, H. Ahmed, a.K., Misk, N.A.a nd Makady, F.M. 1985. The arterial blood supply and venous drainage of the udder in buffaloes (*Bos bubalis* L.). Assuit Vet., Med. J., 14(27): 19-23.

Bali, B.D. 1962. A buffalo cow gives milk without calving. Indian Vet., J., 39: 351-352.

Barnwal, A.K. and Dhingra, L.D. 1978. A note on the lymphatic drainage of mammary gland of buffaloes. Indian J. Anim. Sci., 48: 753-755.

Bhat, P.N. 1979. Genetic parameters of milk production and scope of increasing milk production in buffaloes *vis-à-vis* cattle. Buffalo Reprod. Art. Insem., pp. 129-142. FAO Anim. Prod. Health Paper 13, Rome.

Bhosrekar, M.R. and Nagpaul, P.K. 1971. Type of udders and teats in some Indian milch breeds of cattle and buffaloes as compared to those of crossbred, Indian J. Dairy Sci., 24: 208-211.

Chandiramani, S.V., Gautam, A.N. and Luktuke, S.N. 1966. Continued use of oxytocin in obtaining milk from difficult buffaloes. Indian J. Dairy Sci. 19: 143-145.

Chantalakhana, C. 1979. Performance of swamp, riverine and crosssbred buffaloes in South East Asia. Buffalo Reprod. Art Insem., pp. 143-151. FAO Anim. Prod. Health Paper 13, Rome.

Chowdhary, M.S. and Chaudhary, A.L. 1981. Studies on peak yield and days to attain peak yield in Mehsana and Surti buffaloes. Indian Vet J., 58: 203-207.

D'angelo, A., and De Franciscis, G. 1966. Structural aspects of the udder of buffalo heifers during hormonally induced lactation. Atti Soc. Ital., Sci. Vet., 20: 371-374.

Dassw, P.D., Basu, S.B. and Sharma, K.N.S. 1976. Effect of frequency of milking in Murrah buffaloes. Indian J. Dairy Sci., 29: 113-116.

Dwivedi, J. and Prabhu, S.S. 1970. Studies on supernumerary teats (SNTs) In Indian buffaloes. J. Remout Vet. Corps, Hisar 9(2): 14-18.

El-Sheikh, A.S. and Sultan, Z.A. 1977. Developmental changes in the udder secretory tissue of the Egyptian buffalo. Indian J. Anim. Sci. 47: 630-635.

Fahmy, M.F.A, Morcos, M.B. and Elgafary, M. 1969. A histological study of the teat of the buffalo. Indian vet J., 46: 856-859.

Ferrara, B., Badolato, F., Minieri, L. and De Franciscis, G. 1966a. Preliminary investigations on the possibility of artificially induced lactation in virgin buffalo heifers. I. Treatment with synthetic oestrogen. Athi. Soc., Ital., Sci. Vet., 20: 363-366.

Ferrara, B., De Paolis, P., Intrieri, F. and Rendina, N. 1966b. Preliminary investigations on the possibility of artificially induced lactation in virgin buffalo heifers. I. Treatment with oestrogen, progesterone and chorionic gonadotropin. Athi. Soc., Ital., Sci. Vet., 20: 367-371.

Fischer, H. 1956. Twin buffaloes with hypoplasia of the udder. Berl. Munch. Tierazzil. Wschr., 69: 89-91.

Fischer, H. 1962. A note on fused and supernumerary teats in Murrah buffaloes. J. Malay, Vet., Med., Ass., 3: 110-112.

Gangwar, P.C., Soni, P.L. and Mehta, S.N. 1980. Effect of environmental cooling on certain physiological and milk ejection responses of buffaloes (*Bos bubalis*). Indian J. Nutr. Dietet., 17: 302-308.

Gotsiridze, N. and Kitoshvili, I. 1981. The effectiveness of buffalo breeding, Zhinotnoodstvo, 3: 37-38.

Gotsiridze, N.K. and Saakova, L.I. 1980. Evaluation of udders of machine milked buffaloes. Gruzinskii Zoovt. Uchebno Issled Inst., Tbilisi, USSR.

Gupta, S.C., Gangwar, P.C.a nd Kooner, D.S. 1974. A note on the effect of weaning on letdown time in buffaloes. Indian J. Anim. Sci. 44: 334-336.

Gupta, S.C., Handa, M.C. and Sahoo. G. 1985. Dairy temperament of buffaloes in relation to their milking ability. Indian J. Dairy Sci., 34: 45-48.

Hafez., A. and Naidu, K.N. 1981. Relation of udder size with milk yield in buffloes. Indian J. Dairy Sci., 34: 45-48.

Hanna, A.K., Hassan, A. Yaseen, A. and Baday, A. 1979. The effectiveness of subcutaneously versus intramuscular administration of oxytocin upon removal of residual milk in buffaloes and cattle., Alexandria J. Agric. Res., 27: 567-574.

Hossain, M.I., Mia, M.A., Khan, M.A.B. and Talukdar, A.H. 1980. The arterial blood supply to the mammary gland of water buffalo. Bangladesh Vet. J., 14: 25-27.

Jadhav, D.S. and Khambata, F.S. 1967. Preliminary observations on complementary milk in a buffalo cow. Indian Vet. J. 782-785.

Kapoor, M. and Ludri, R.S. 1984. Effect of different milking intervals in buffaloe on secretion rates of milk and some of its organic constitutents. Indian J. Anim. Sci. , 54: 153-157.

Katiyar, R.S. and Chandra, G. 1983a. Morphology of suspensary apparatus in buffalo udder. Indian Vet. J., 60: 347-349.

Katiyar, R.S. and Chandra, G. 1983b. Arterial system in udder of buffalo (*Bubalus bubalis*). Indian Vet. J., 60: 70-9-713.

Kumar, R. and Bhat, P.N. 1979. Lactation curve in Indian buffaloes. Indian J. Dairy Sci., 32: 156-160.

Ludri, R.S. 1980. Milk letdown response and residual milk in buffaloes. Indian J. Anim. Sci. 50: 891-893.

Ludri, R.S. and Sarma, P.A. 1981. Supernumerary teats in crossbred cows and buffaloes. Indian J. Dairy Sci., 34: 252-353.

Malossini, F. 1967. Variation in the produciotn of milk and its constituents during lactation and their relationship in buffalo cows. Annali Inst. Sper. Zootec. Roma, 11: 91-121.

Mangurkar, B.R. and Desai, R.N. 1981. Udder measurements and their relationship with selection index values in buffaloe Indian Vet. J., 58: 392-395.

Maqsood, M. 1956. Galactopoetic action of thyroxine in cattle kept in subtropical countries. Agric. Pakistan, 7: 77-82.

Maymone, B. 1945. Buffalo breeding in Italy. Z. Tierz. Zuchtbiol, 52: 1-44.

Minier, L., Intrieri, F. and Romano, M. 1966. Investigations on the chemical composition of the mammary secretion of virgin buffalo heifers during hormonally induced lactation. Att., Soc. Ital., Sci., Vet., 30: 374-378.

Moussa, M.H.G. 1982. Micromopholocial study of the blood vessels of the teat of buffalo (*Bos bubalis*, L.) in Egypt. Anatomischer Anzeiger, 152: 129-140.

Nosier, M.B. 1972. Relationship between milk yield and glandular tissue within artificially developed mammary gland of buffalo heifer. Egyptian J. Vet. Sci., 9: 81-85.

Nosier, M.B> Shalash, M.R., Zaki, K.M. and Afiefy, M.N. 1973. Some aspects of lactation in buffalo. Atti del VII Simposio Inter. Di. Zooteenia, Milano. April 15-17., 1972.

Olenov, Yu.M. 1954. Causes for the differences between the butter fat content of portions of milk obtained after milking. Doki, Akad. Nauk., SSR. 97(2): 361-364.

Patton, S. 1969. Milk., Sci. Amer., 221-58.

Pandey, H.S., Kumar, S. and Katpatal., B.G. 1981. Note on proportionate and actual milk yield from individual quarters of udder in murrah buffaloes. Indian J. Anim Sci., 51: 105-107.

Polikhrono, D. and TOsev, A. 1970. Functional characters of udder quarters in local buffaloes. Zhivot. Nauk, 7(3): 11-15.

Ragab, M.T. 1979. Buffaloes in the middle east for milk and meat production Buffalo Repord. Art. Insem., pp.1 55-162. FAO Anim. Prod. Health paper 13, Rome.

Ragab, M.T., Shafie, M.M.and Kilani, M. 1971. Milk yield and milking rates of the individual quarters of the udder in buffaloes, Egyptian cows and Friesian cows. J. Anim. Prod., UAR, 9: 67-78.

Rao, A.V.N. and Murthy, T.S. 1984. Indicience of udder and teat anomalies in buffaloes. Indian vet.J., 61: 311-314.

Rao, A.V.N., Sreemannarayan, O. and Rao, P.V. 1982. Hormonal induction of lactation in buffalo heifers. Livestock Advisor, 7(12): 29-31.

Roy, P.K. and Nagpaul, P.K. 1984a. Influence of genetic and non-genetic factors on temperament score and other traits of dairy management. Indian J. Anim. Sci., 54: 566-567.

Roy, P.K. and Nagpaul, P.K. 1984b., Studies on effect of temperament score on different traits in dairy animals. Indian J. Dairy Sci., 37: 74-75.

Saakova, L.I. 1979a. Testing and evaluating milk rates in buffaloes. Trudy. Gruz, Zootekh Vet Nauchno. Issled. Inst., 108(42): 141-144.

Saxena, H.K. 1973. Variation in shape and size of udder in murrah buffaloes. Indian J. Anim. Sci., 43: 468-471.

Saxena, S.C. and Prabhu, S.S. 1970. Relation between udder an dteat traits and milk yield in Indian buffaloes. Indian J. Anim. Prod., 1: 97-100.

Saxena, S.C. and Prabhu, S.S. 1972. Variation in udder size and udder indices of Indian bufflaoes. Indian J. Anim. Prod., 2: 1-4.

Shafie, M.M., Ragab, M.T. and Kilay, M. 1969. Milking time and initial milk yield in buffaloes, Egyptian cattle and Friesian cattle. J. Anim. Prod. UAR, 9: 211-219.

Shalash, M.R., Salama, A.A. and Moursi, H. 1961a. Trials on the artificial induction of lactation in buffaloes. Proc., VIII Intern., Cong. Anim. Prod., Hungary, 1: 217.

Shalash, M.R., Salama, A.A. and El Guindi, M. 1961b. Note on artificial induction of lactation in buffaloes.Emp. J. Exp. Agric., 29: 45-48.

Shalash, M.R., Salama, A., Nawito, N. and Mousa, A. 1964. Artificial induction of lactation in relation to reproductive efficiency in buffaloes. Proc., 5th Int. Cong. Anim. Reprode. AI, Trento, II: 250-262.

Sidhu, M.S. and Pal, R.N. 1978. Studies on the effect of lactation number and stage of lactation on some physical characteristics in Murrah buffaloes. Haryana Agric., Univ. J. Res., 8: 131-135.

Singh, M. and Bhatnagar, D.S. 1977. Size and shape of udder and teats I brown Swiss corssbreds vis-à-vis zebu cows and Murrah buffaloes. Indian Vet. J., 54: 377-383.

Soni, P.L. 1975. M.Sc. Thesis, Punjab Agric. University, Ludhiana.

Sud, S.C. 1979. A note on hormonal induction of lactation in buffaloes. Indian J. Anim. Sci., 49: 229-231.

Sud, S.C. and Singh, R.V. 1974. A note on the development of udder and induction of lactation in young buffaloes. Indian J. Anim. Sci., 44: 335-336.

Taneja, G.C. and Bhatnagar, D.S. 1958. Qualitative and quantitative variations in the milkyield 1. Relationship between udder score and milk yield. J. Vet. Anim. Husb., Res., MHOW, 3: 86-89.

Tripathi, M.D. and Saraswati, B.L. 1982. Qualitative and quantitative variations in the milk from different quarters of udder of buffaloes. Asian J. Diary Res., 1: 227-230.

Tsankova, M. 1983. Phenotipic correlations between udder measurement sand the lactation milkyield in buffalo crossbreds and back crosses. Zhivortnov'dni Nauki, 20(5): 39-44.

Tsankova, M. and Tosev, A. 1980. Some functional udder characteristics of female buffaloes, crosses of local Bugarian with Murrah buffaloes. Zhivotonov' dni Nauki, 217(7): 16-22.

Turabov, T. 1982. Evaluation of milk production of female Caucasian buffaloes. Molochne i. Myasnoe Skotovodstve, 5: 19-22.

Turabov, T. and Abllaev, M.G. 1979. Evaluation of udder so female Caucasian buffaloes on milkability (Preliminary communication. Molochne i. Myasnoe Skotovodstve.

Verma, G.S., Tomer, S.S. and Tomer, O.S. 1984. Indicence of supernumerary tests (SNT) and their relationship with some economic traits in Murrah buffaloes. Indian Vet., J., 61: 521-522.

□□□

4

Buffalo Milk and Milk Products

Buffalo is a triple purpose animal providing milk, power and meat for human requirements. The primary contribution of riverine breeds is the milk production, while swamp buffaloes are the famous draught animals in the paddy growing countries. All types of buffaloes are slaughtered for meat production normally after their utilization as milch draught animals intensive fattening for meat production is practiced in some Mediterranean countries of Europe and Asia, Egypt, Brazil, West Indies. Thailand and Philippines etc.

Milk

Milk is the normal secretion of mammary glands, secreted after parturition for the nourishment of the new born calves. It is fluid complex system presenting different phases viz. (i) Continuous phase consisting of water and water soluble milk constituents like lactose, slat and water soluble vitamins etc. (ii) Colloidal phase consisting of minute particles of casein, albumin, globulins and enzymes dispersion. And (iii) Emulsion phase consisting of larger globules of milk fat, phospholipids, cholesterol, fat soluble vitamins and small quantity of associated minerals in the form of organic compounds.

Whole milk: Normal milk secretion of a healthy udder after about 7-10 days of calving is known as whole milk.

Separated or skim milk: the fluid milk residue left after the removal of cream is known as separated or skim milk. It contains about 0.1 per cent milk fat.

Standardized milk: the adjustment of milk fat and/or solids not fat percentage of milk according to prevention of Food Adulteration (PFA) rules is known as the standardization of milk. This is done by the addition of skim milk in case of high fat milk and fresh cream in case of low milk. The amount of skim milk of fresh cream required to obtain the desired fat percentage in milk is calculated by the Pearson's square on weight basis.

Example 1. Determination of the amount of 40% fresh cream to be missed in 5% whole milk to prepare a standardized milk of 6% milk fat content

Calculations

Cream	40	1
Milk	5	34

Answer: A mixture of 1 kg fresh cream (40% fat) and 34 kg milk (5% fat) will give a standardized milk of 6% fat content.

Example 2. Determination of quantity of 0.1% skim milk for mixing with 7% whole milk to standardize for 6% fat content

Calculations

Skim milk	0.1%	1
Whole milk	7%	5.9

Answer: A mixture of 1 kg skim milk and 5.9 milk will provide a standardized milk of 6% fat content.

Homogenized milk: The whole milk processed in a homogenizer for reducing the size of fat globules to such an extent that no apparent layer of cream appears on the surface of milk even after 48 hours undisturbed storage. The size of fat globules in homogenized milk is mostly less than 2 microns in diameter. Homogenization of milk is affected by two factors i.e. (i) the temperature of homogenization which should be preferably 65-70°C. A temperature range of 38-49°C should be avoided during and after homogenization to control the lipase activity in the milk, (ii) pressure of homogenization- a single stage pressure of 2000-2500 psi is adequate for the homogenization of milk containing less than 6 percent milk fat. For higher fat percentage, two stage homogenization is required in first stage pressure is maintained at 2000 psi followed by 500 psi in the second stage.

Toned milk: The milk containing 3 percent milk fat and 8.5 per cent solids not fat obtained by mixing water and skim milk powder in whole milk is known as tonned or single toned milk.

Double toned milk: The milk adjusted with the addition of water and skim milk powder to contain 1.5 per cent milk fat and 9 per cent solids not fat is known as double toned milk.

Humanized milk: The modification of buffalo milk through the addition of water, sugar and/or skim milk powder to resemble the human milk in chemical composition is known as the humanization of buffalo milk and the milk thus obtained is called humanized milk.

Reconstituted milk: The fluid milk prepared by dispersing whole milk powder in water in the ratio of 1:7 or 1:8 is known as reconstituted milk. Spray dried milk powder is preferred for the preparation of reconstituted or rehydrated milk because it is more soluble and leaves little sediment.

Recombined milk: The fluid milk prepared by the mixing of butter ft, skim milk powder and water in the proportion present in whole milk or toned milk.

Sterilized milk: The milk heated at 100-110°C for about 30 minutes is known as sterilized milk. The sterilized milk has longer storage life at room temperature and it is free from the pathogenic and other harmful microorganisms-except the heat resistant spore forming bacteria, if any, present in the raw milk. Sterilization of milk result from significant loss of vitamin C and B complex.

Pasteurized milk: The fluid milk heated at 63°C or 145°F for 30 minutes or at 72°C (161°F) for 15 seconds and then quickly cooled below 5°C (41°F) is known as pasteurized milk. The pasteurization of milk is common practice in the organized dairies for the supply of safe milk for human consumption.

Market milk: The whole milk sold to consumers is usually called as market milk. It may be milk of a single cow or buffalo, a cow herd, buffalo herd or mixed whole milk of cows and buffaloes.

Composition of Buffalo Milk

The constituents of buffalo milk are similar to normal mammalian milk. Main constituents of whole milk are water, milk, fat, protein, factose and inorganic matter or ash. The composition of milk in diary terminology is given as milk-fat, total solids, solids-not fat and ash. The other components of milk are phospholipids, sterols, enzymes, vitamins, pigments and dissolved gases (Ling, 1948). The various constituents of milk may be illustrated as follows (Table 4.1).

Table 4.1. Various milk constituents

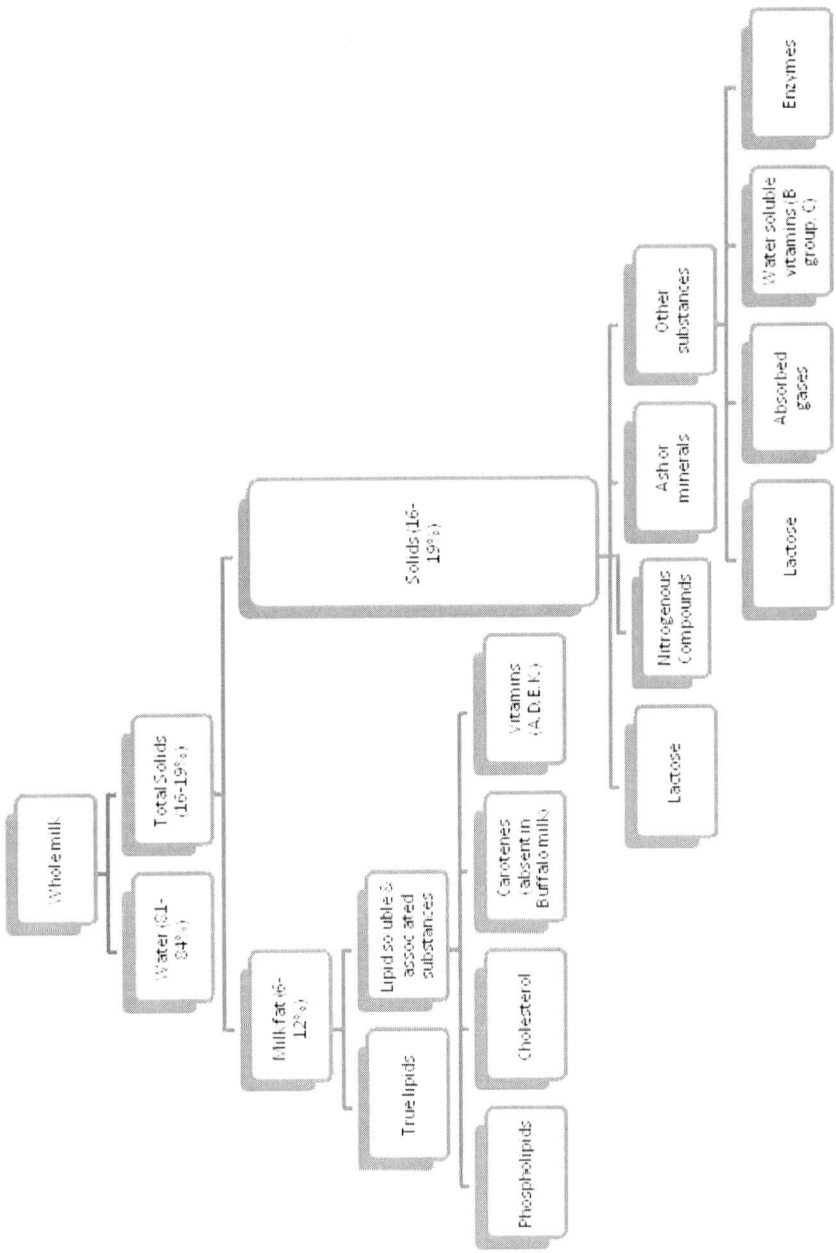

Chemical composition of Buffalo Milk

The average chemical composition of milk of different types of buffaloes shows significant variations (Table 1). The milk fat is most variable component of the milk, which is normally higher in draught type swamp buffaloes than the dairy type riverine buffaloes except the Bhadawari breed found in the south-east parts of Uttar Pradesh and adjoining areas of Madhya Pradesh in India.

Factors affecting the chemical composition of milk: The chemical composition of milk is quite variable and it is influenced by several factors. The milk constituents are almost common but their proportion differ significantly between the animals. The variation decrease with the increase in the size of herd and greatest variation is observed in the fat percentage of milk. The following factors are found to be responsible for the differences in the chemical composition of milk.

1. **Variation due to breed and type:** Great variation in chemical of the buffalo milk of different genetic groups is apparent in Table 2. Such difference is also found in different breeds of buffalo from the same agro-climatic condition (Table. 4.2). The chemical composition of milk is relatively less variable between the breeds of same place (Rao and nagarcenkar, 1977; Sharma *et al.,* 1980).

Table 4.2 Variation in milk composition due to types of breeds

Types of breeds	Milk composition (%)					
	Total solids	Fat	Protein	Lactose	Solids not fat	Ash
Indian river buffaloes						
Murrah	17.0	6.9	4.1	5.1	10.4	0.9
Bhadawari	19.9	10.5	4.2	5.2	9.4	1.0
Indian Swamp buffaloes						
Assamese Manipuri		7.5	4.1	5.6	9.8	0.9
Egyptian dairy buffalo		6.4	3.9	5.8	10.0	0.9
Vietnamese		8.2	4.1	5.6	10.1	0.9

2. **Variation due to stage of lactation:** Almost all milk constituents are significantly affected by the stage of lactation. Milk fat, protein and casein percentage increases while lactose decreases with the

progress in lactation period (Table 4.3). The various milk constituents normally decline in early lactation upto peak yield and thereafter shows a rising trend (Basu *et al.*, 1948; Singh *et al.*, 1961; Salerno, 1967; Kumar *et al.*, 1980). Most of the milk constituents showed inconsistent monthly variation in the Egyptian buffaloes (Abd El-Salam and Shibiny, 10/966) but definite trend (Table 4.4) in Murrah buffaloes (Pandey, 1981).

Table 4.3 Composition of milk during different stages of lactation.

Stage of lactation	Fat	Protein	Casein	Lactose
Early lactation	6.8	3.61	2.94	5.11
Mid lactation	7.0	3.67	3.01	5.09
Late lactation	8.4	3.91	3.15	4.84

Table 4.4 Monthly variation in milk composition

Month of lactation	Egyptian Buffalo			Murrah Buffalo		
	Fat	Protein	Lactose	Fat	Protein	Lactose
1	6.16	3.69	5.30	6.19	4.61	4.66
2	5.73	3.75	5.03	5.80	4.20	4.66
3	6.59	3.59	5.18	6.12	4.13	4.66
4	5.57	3.51	5.00	6.46	4.06	4.76
5	6.11	3.88	5.16	6.56	4.08	4.63
6	7.20	3.73	4.86	6.86	4.08	4.63
7	7.05	3.59	4.68	7.00	4.09	4.85
8	7.98	4.34	5.00	7.53	4.26	4.69
9	7.01	3.53	5.11	8.06	4.39	4.72
10	-	-	-	8.16	4.45	4.75
11	7.18	4.05	4.64	-	-	-

3. **Variation due to parity:** Variable repots are available on the effect of parity on the chemical composition of milk. The various milk constituents are generally low (Table 4.5) in the first calvers of Egyptian and Indian buffaloes (Ragab *et al.*, 1958; Asker *et al.*, 1971; Pandey, 1981), whereas higher percentage of milk constituents are observed in the Russain buffaloes (Akhundov, 1966, Dzaforov, 1969).

Table 4.5. Variation in milk composition due to parity

Parity	Fat (%)	Protein (%)	Total Solids (%)	Solids-not fat (%)
Egyptian buffalo				
First	6.21	3.81	16.17	9.96
Second	6.38	3.91	16.42	10.04
Third	6.41	3.86	16.43	10.02
Murrah Buffaloes				
First	6.76	4.07	16.74	9.98
Second	6.84	4.19	16.83	9.99
Third	6.74	4.20	16.69	9.95
Fourth	6.95	4.35	16.96	10.01
Fifth	7.08	4.37	17.09	10.01
Russian Buffalo				
First	8.75	4.52	18.52	9.77
Second	871	4.47	18.40	9.78
Third	8.69	4.41	17.83	9.14

4. **Variation due to season:** Seasonal variation in milk composition is associated with the change in agro-climatic conditions affecting the chemical composition of the feeds and fodders. Significant seasonal variation in milk composition may be observed (Table 4.6), but the trend will differ due to breed and location (El-Shokkary and Hassan, 1949, Ghosh and Anantakrishnan, 1963; Khan *et al.,* 1970; El-Ghandour *et al.,* 1979).

Table 4.6 Seasonal variation in milk composition (%)

Season	Fat	Solids-not fat	Protein	Lactose+Ash
Winter	6.75	9.67	3.97	5.69
Summer	6.49	9.67	3.88	5.79
South-west monsoon	7.09	9.52	3.87	5.67
North-east mansoon	6.81	9.66	3.95	5.70

5. **Variation due to pregnancy:** Pregnancy has significant effect on the milk composition probably due to demand of nutrients for foetal development. Pregnancy affected the various milk constituents and a definite trend of increase in lactose percentage and fall in ash percentage (Table 4.7) has been reported during the rising a well as declining phases of the lactation period (Parekh and Gangwar, 1968).

Table 4.7. Variation in milk composition due to pregnancy

Milk composition (%)	Non pregnant	Early pregnancy	Mid pregnancy	Late pregnancy
Rising phase of lactation period				
Fat	6.10	6.68	6.99	-
Total solids	16.50	17.01	17.39	-
Solids-not fat	10.40	10.33	10.99	-
Protein	4.57	4.46	4.79	-
Lactose	4.83	5.14	5.40	-
Ash	6.81	0.73	0.71	-
Declining phase of lactation period				
Fat	7.13	7.87	7.77	7.47
Total solids	17.45	18.54	18.24	18.25
Solids-not fat	10.32	10.65	10.47	10.78
Protein	4.74	4.76	4.53	4.76
Lactose	4.73	5.12	0.63	0.48
Ash	0.85	0.77	0.63	0.48

6. **Diurnal variation:** Diural variation in milk composition is frequently observed. Usually higher percentage of total solids and milk fat associated with lower milk yield at the evening milk than the morning milk I squite common in buffaloes (Fahmey, 1974; Dash and Basu, 1975; El-Ghandour *et al.*, 1979). However, such variations are not consistent and differ between the farms (Table 4.8). Variation in milk fat percentage is normally highest amongst all the milk constituents (Pandey, 1961).

Table 4.8. Diurnal variation in milk composition (%)

Farm/Herd	Fat		Protein		Lactose		Total solids	
	M	E	M	E	M	E	M	E
Izatnagar	7.81	7.16	4.45	4.39	4.75	4.73	18.09	17.04
Pantnagar	7.25	7.29	4.39	4.35	4.64	4.65	17.27	17.27
Manjhra	6.39	6.24	4.03	4.04	4.77	4.74	16.32	16.20
Chak-Ganjaria	6.84	6.45	4.11	4.11	4.60	4.57	16.61	16.26
Pooled milk	6.94	6.60	4.19	4.16	4.68	4.66	16.87	16.49

7. **Variation due to season of calving:** Difference in milk composition is observed duet to season of calving (Table 4.9). The percentage of various milk constituents of Egyptian buffaloes are higher in summer calves than in winter calves (Ragab *et al.*, 1974). In Murrah buffaloes, the milk of winter calvers is generally richer than the summer and monsoon calvers (Pandey, 1981).

Table 4.9. Variation in milk composition due to pregnancy

Season calving	Fat (%)	Total solids(%)	Solids not fat (%)	Protein (%)
Egyptian buffaloes				
Winter	6.30	16.33	10.03	3.89
Summer	6.52	16.62	10.10	3.90
Murrah buffaloes				
Winter	709	17.21	10.07	4.24
Summer	7.49	17.60	10.06	4.42
Monsoon	7.11	17.15	9.98	4.32

8. **Variation due to milking portion:** Significant variation occurs in the composition of different portions of milk at the milking time and fat percentage is usually high in the last fraction of milk and the residual milk obtained after stripping at the end of milking (Olenov, 1954; El-Shazly *et al.*, 1974; Hanna *et al.*, 1979; Ludri, 1980). Fat percentage in different portions of milk may show more variation in the first month of lactation period (Table 4.10). Large variation occurs in the fat and total solids content of residual milk (Table 4.11).

Table 4.10. Difference in fat percentage of different portions of milk

Portion of milk	Month of lactation		
	Ist	4th	7th
1	5.61	9.59	9.10
2	4.86	7.52	10.60
3	7.04	9.50	17.40
4	10.76	11.20	14.61

Table 4.11. Difference in composition of normal and residual milk

Constituents (%)	Normal milk		Residual milk	
	Range	Mean	Range	Mean
Milk fat	3.7-7.6	5.9	4.8-22.0	12.15
Total solids	13.2-18.3	16.0	14.2-32.4	22.20
Solids not fat	9.4-11.1	10.1	9.4-11.01	10.05

9. **Variation due to milking interval or frequency of daily milking:** Frequency of daily milking affects milks composition (Table 4.12) but the variation in composition does not show a definite trend (Dass *et al.*, 1976; Kapoor and Ludri, 1984).

Table 4.12. Variation in milk composition due to milking interval

Milk constituents (%)	Milking interval (hr)			
	4	8	12	16
Milk fat	6.82	7.04	6.87	7.06
Total solids	17.33	17.22	17.30	17.51
Solids not fat	10.46	10.37	10.40	10.45
Protein	4.43	4.42	4.43	4.33
Lactose	4.58	4.64	4.61	4.75

10. **Variation due to udder massage before milking:** Light massage of udder before milking increases milk yield as well as fat percentage in milk (Alim *et al.*, 1977; Gotsiridze and Kitoshvili, 1981). The effect of udder massage on milk composition is quite variable (Table. 4.13).

Table 4.13. Difference in fat percentage of different portions of milk

Milk components	Wet massage with warm cloth	Dry hand massage
Milk fat	6.88±0.76	6.39a"0.75
Total solids	16.25±0.98	15.78+1.24
Solids not fat	9.38±0.42	9.39±0.45

11. **Variation due to udder quarters:** Milk composition of different udder quarters of the same buffalo (Table 4.14) differs significantly (Polikhronov and Tosev, 1970).

Table 4.14. Variation due to udder quarters.

Milk constituents	Left fore	Right fore	Left rear	Right rear
Milk yield (%)	20.61	21.23	29.77	28.29
Fat in milk	8.38	8.27	8.34	8.34

12. **Variation due to lactation milk yield:** a negative correlation is normally found between the milk yield and percentage of fat, protein and total solids of the milk (El-Ghandour *et al.,* 1980).

13. **Variation due to environmental cooling:** Arrangement of environmental cooling for the amelioration of heat stress significantly increase the daily milk yield. The increase in milk yield has been found to be associated with the fall in fat percentage and increase in lactose percentage of milk (Table 4.15). The effect of cooling arrangement is almost similar during the rising and declining phases of lactation period (Soni *et al.,* 1980).

Table 4.15. Variation in milk composition due to environmental cooling.

Treatments	Milk yield (Kg/day)	Fat (%)	Lactose (%)
Lactation phase I			
Control	7.5	7.59	4.26
Shower bath	7.6	7.65	4.45
Wallowing 8.5	7.43	4.58	4.58
Lactation phase II			
Control	6.8	7.96	4.40
Shower bath	7.0	7.98	4.52
Wallowing 8.5	7.3	7.70	4.77

14. **Variation due to individual, herd, families and lines of buffaloes:** Variation in the composition of milk due to individuals, herds or farms, families and lines is not uncommon (El-SOkkary and Hassan, 1949, Dzhafarov, 1971; Pandey, 1981). The variation is greater due to individuality of the animals (Table 4.16).

Table 4.15.

Factors	Fat (%)	Total Solids (%)	Protein (%)
Individual	4.25-10.20 (6.64)		2.69-5.05 (3.92)
Herd	5.50-7.50 (6.60)		3.54-4.40 (3.96)
Family A	8.72	18.28	4.46
Family B	9.40	18.37	4.51
Line I	9.07	18.78	4.86
Line II	8.49	17.91	4.42
Line II	8.30	17.80	4.50

15. **Variation due to feeds:** The composition of rations and plane of nutrition may significantly affect the milk composition. Feeding of green leguminous fodders increases milk yield of less fat content (Pandey *et al.,* 1969). Additional feeding of concentrates over the requirement may not affect the milk composition (Touny *et al.,* 1976; Kumar and Tripathi, 1978) but significant cut in concentrate feeds ona wheat bhoosa based diet may cause considerable fall in milk yield but increase in fat content (Shukla *et al.,* 1972). Feeding of oil in diets affects the content and compositon of fat in milk (Ahuja *et al.,* 1972).

Milk Distribution Systems

One or more of the following activities are involved milk distribution systems:

1. Milk Production
2. Purchase and collection of milk
3. Preservation and transportation of milk
4. Sterilization pasteurization of milk
5. Packaging of milk
6. Distribution of milk

Milk production: The milk produces may be classified into three groups i.e. (i) rural milk producers comprising farmers of different economic classes and landless farm families, (ii) urban and sub-urban dairy owners maintaining small to medium sized herds of lactation buffaloes (iii) organized daily farms of Government institutions, Co-operative Societies and Private organizations.

Purchase and collection of milk: The milk is purchased by retain consumers, Middleman, halwais, milk cooperatives and processing factories. The milk collection system differs in different areas. Mostly middleman or a dudhias collect milk from door to door or at a common place according to convenience, while milk cooperatives establish milk collection centres with a small laboratory facility for milk testing, preferably milk fat percentage for the determination of milk price. Price of milk is normally paid in cash and/or kid at the milk collection centres according to fat percentage in the milk. The payment may weekly, fortnightly or monthly. Halais in the Indian subcontinent mostly prefer to purchase milk on the basis of khoa recovery.

Preservation and transportation of milk: Milk is preserved by the use of common preservatives like hydrogen peroxide and cooling with the help of a water soaked jute patti on the metallic milk containers and by chilling, if chilling plant is available.

Normally milk is transported twice daily to market, milk collection centres and the milk processing plants. The mode of transport depends on the amount of milk, distance, transport facilities and local conditions. Milk may be transported by road, rail and water routes (Table 4.17).

Table 4.17. Modes of milk transportation.

Mode	Quantity of milk (kg)	Distance (km)
Road Transports		
Head load	10-30	Upto 10
Bahangi/shoulder sling	10-50	Upto 10
Pack animals		
Bullock	40-60	Upto 10
Pony	40-60	Upto 20
Camel	40-60	Upto 15
Bullock cart	200-400	Upto 10
Tonga/Ekka	200-300	Upto 20
Bicycle	50-60	Upto 30
Rickshaw	100-200	Upto 25
Auto rickshaw	100-200	Upto 25
Truck/Tankers	½ - 5 ton	More than 50

Water routes		
Boats		
Steamers		
Rail transport		
Common containers	25-100	Upto 50
Milk carriage	10 tons cap.	Long distance

Different types of containers are used for the transporation of fluid milk and their selection depends on the amount of milk, distance of transportation, initial cost of containers, working life of the containers, mode of transportation, easiness of cleaning and availability etc. The following types of containers are commonly used for the transportation of milk.

1. Baked earthenwares
2. Wooden cans
3. Hollow bamboo cylinders
4. Aluminium cans
5. Galvanized iron cans
6. Empty tin containers available after the disposal fo vegetable oils
7. Plastic containers
8. Motor driven or rail tankers with arrangement for milk chilling.

Sterilization and pasteurization: For increasing the keeping quality of fluid milk it is essential to remove or reduce its microbial content. Milk is mad efree from microorganisms through sterilization and microbial count is significantly reduced and their multiplication is controlled through the pasteurization. The surplus fluid milk of evening milk is normally boiled and either kept for sale in next morning or cultured for dahi making. This practice is followed by small milk producers of remote areas. The pasteurization of milk is practiced in the organize dairies.

Packaging of fluid milk: The pasteurized milk is filled in sterilized clean glass bottles or disposable paper/plastic containers of 0.5, 1, 2 and 5 litres capacity and packed in cartons for retail sale. Bulk milk packaging may done in alloy or plastic containers.

Distribution of milk: The distribution of milk may be very simple like retails sale to consumers at the unorganized dairy farms of urban areas or a complex system of collection, processing, standardization, pasteurization, packaging and distribution process of the organized dairies. Following are the common milk distribution systems:

i) **Direct retail sale of fluid milk at eh place of production:** It is a daily routine sale for 1-2 hours in morning and evening at the time of milk. The requirement of consumers varies from quarter litre to 4-5 litres daily.

ii) **Door delivery:** Fresh fluid milk is sold from door to door within 1-3 hours of production. The vendors may be either producer or a middleman.

iii) **Bulk supply to shops:** The milk collected by middle man from the rural areas is sold to shops in bulk. Average daily requirement of shops varies from 10 to 100 kg or more depending upon the market requirement of milk and milk products.

iv) **Supply of pasteurized milk through booth or sale agents:** This system is common in cities and towns having organized dairies. The milk is available in a half or one litre sealed containers. The mode of sale may be cash payment or coupon system. The third and most convenient system is the machine delivery where fixed quantity of milk is delivered by the automatic machine against pushing the cost of milk in definite coins. However, procurement of coins is a limiting factors in this system.

Milk Products

Various kinds of milk products are quite popular in the human dietary since ages. Buffalo milk is preferred over cow milk due to its high fat and total solids contents for the preparation of several milk products of the tropical and other buffalo breeding countries. Approximately half of the total milk produced in India is believed to be utilized for the production of various dairy products which are more remunerative than the sale of fluid milk. The various milk products may be classified into the followings six groups:

1. Fluid milk products
2. Condensed milk products
3. Dried or dehydrated milk products

4. Coagulated milk products
5. Fermented or cultured milk products, and
6. Products of the cream, butter and ghee industry

Fluid milk products: The milk products flavoured and sweetened for increasing the palatability and containing milk fat not less than the minimum legal requirement of milk are known as milks, while those with low fat content are known as drinks (milk drinks). The common examples are chocolate milk, fruit flavoured milk and vitaminized milk etc. the most popular fluid milk drink is milk shake. These products are normally coloured, sterilized and bottles in hygienic conditions and used for cold drinks during the summer season.

Condensed milk products: The milk products prepared by partial evaporation of water through the heating of whole milk, partially separated milk and skim milk are known as condensed milks. They may or may not contain added sugars (Sucrose). The different kinds of condensed milks are described as follows:

i) **Unsweetened condensed milk/ partial evaporated milk:** The milk products manufactured by the partial removal of water through heating is called unsweetened condensed milk or partial evaporated milk. It may contain not more than 0.3 per cent of calcium chloride, citric acid, sodium nitrate or sodium salt of orthophosphoric acid or poly phosphoric acid in the final products. Unsweetened condensed milk should contain not less than 8 per cent milk fat and 26 per cent milk solids not fat. Buffalo milk needs standardization of milk fat through the addition of skim milk for the manufacture of unsweetened condensed milk according to the legal standards.

ii) **Unsweetened condensed skim milk:** Unsweetened condensed skim milk is manufactured by partial evaporation of moisture of separated milk through heat treatment. The addition of calcium chloride, citric acid, sodium citrate and sodium salt salts of orthophsophoric acid or polyphosphoric acid should not exceed 0.3 per cent by weight of the final product. It should not contain more than 0.5 percent milk fat and less than 20 per cent total milk solids.

iii) **Sweetened condensed milk:** The whole milk or standardized milk condensed through the partial evaporation of moisture content by heat treatment under a high vaccum after the addition of cane sugar should not contain less than 9 per cent milk fat, 31 per cent total milk solids and 40 percent added sugar (sucrose). The preservatives concentration as mentioned for the unsweetened condensed milk should not be more than 03 per cent by weight of the finished product.

iv) **Sweetened condensed skim milk:** It is prepared by partial evaporation of moisture of skimmed milk and addition of sugar (sucrose). The various preservatives as mentioned for the unsweetened condensed milk should not exceed 0.3 per cent by weight of the finished product. The milk fat should not more than 0.5 percent, total mok solids less than 26 per cent and cane sugar less than 40 per cent by weight.

The specification for sweetened condensed milks approved by the Indian standards Institution (IS, 1166 of 1973) are given in (Table 4.18).

Table 4.18 ISI (BIS) specification for sweetened condensed milks

Charactristics	Whole milk	Skimmed milk
Total milk solids (%), Min	31.0	26.0
Milk fat (%), Min	9.0	0.5 Max.
Sucrose (%), Min	400	40.0
Acidity as lactic acid (%), Max.	0.35	0.35
Total bacterial count per g, Max.	500	500
Coliform count per g	Nil	Nil
Yeast and mould count per g. Max.	10	10

Uses of condensed milk: Condensed milk is prepared mainly for use in the remote areas where regular supply of fluid milk is not assured. Condensation and other treatments increase its keeping quality and facilitate easy transportation when packed air tight after sterilization. The common uses are as follows:

i) Preparation of reconstituted milk

ii) Preparation of milk containing beverages like tea and coffee, etc.

iii) Preparation of milk foods like kheer, ice cream, kulfi and other sweets.

Dried milk products: The milk products manufactured by the evaporation of moisture by heat treatment or other means are dried milks or milk powder, Milk powder contains less than 5 per cent moisture by weight. It may be whole milk powder or skimmed milk powder. The content of various additives like calcium chloride, citric acid, sodium citrate and sodium salt of orthophosphoric or polyphosphoric acid should not be more than 0.3 per cent and that of butylated hydroxyl anisole 0.01 per cent by weight of the finished product. Whole milk powder hydroxyl anisole 0.01 per cent by weight of the finshed product. Whole milk powder shold not contain less than 26 per cent milk fat and skim milk powder may not contain higher than 1.5 per cent milk fat. The total acidity expressed as lactic acid should be below 1.2 per cent in whole milk powder and 1.5 per cent in skim milk powder. The standard bacterial count (plate count) should not be more than 50000 per gm and coliform bacterial count higher than 90 per g. maximum solubility index should be 15 and 2 for the roller dried and spary dried milk powders, respectively as per the PFA Rules (1976) in India.

Uses of dried milk or milk powder

i) For preparation of reconstituted milk

ii) For preparation of tea and coffee

iii) For the preparation of cultured milk products and sweet dishes containing milk as ain ingredient.

Coagulated milk products: Raw or heated milk is coagulated by the addition of citric acid, lemon juice, lactic acid or sour whey. The coagulum thus obtained is strained and processed for the preparation of chana, paneer, cheese and their products.

Fermented or cultured milk products: The main products prepared from raw or heat milk with the help of natural or specific bacteria culture are known as fermented or cultured milk products. Common products are dahi (curd), yoghurt and chakka (Srikhand) etc.

Concentrated butter fat products or the products of cream, butter and ghee industry: Common milk products containing higher percentage of milk fat prepared through physical processing are cream, butter, makkhan and ghee/samna.

Common Milk products

Various common milk products prepared from buffalo milk in different countries are ghee or samna (classified butter or butter oil), cream, butter, cheese and fermented milk products like dahi and yoghurt. Several varieties of cheese are prepared indifferent countries and some of the popular varieties are given in (Table 4.19).

Table 4.19. Popular cheeses of buffalo milk in different countries.

Name of cheese	Country
Domiati	Egypt
Karish	Egypt
Mis/Mish	Egypt
Ras	Egypt
Roomy	Egypt
Providone	Egypt/Italy
Mozrella	Italy
Shankalish	Syria
Feta	Greece
Teleme	Egypt/Greece
Salamora	Bulgaria
Brandza de Braila	Romania
Cheddar	India, Egypt, Italy etc.
Ricotta	Italy
Grouda	Dutch

1. **Domiati cheese:** it is one of the most popular cheeses of Egypt and it is also known in other Arabian countries. Unlike other pickled cheeses, the domiati cheese is prepared from the salted milk. Domiati cheese is prepared from whole milk of buffalo or cow or a mixture of hole and skim milk in different ratios. However, buffalo milk is preferred due to its high fat content for the production of rich domiati cheese.

About 5-15 per cent finely powdered salt is added directly in the raw milk. It is used to control the microbial growth during the manufacture of cheese at a relatively high temperature. The salt milk is strained through a piece of muslin or cheese cloth to clean it from visible impurities. The strained milk is heated before renneting by one of the following three methods:

i) Direct warming to 35-40°C or 95-105°F.

ii) Heating for 15 minutes at 65oC (150°F) and then cooling to 35-40°C. This process sis helpful in siginficatn reduction of bacteria count, avoidance of gas holes in the cheese and improvement of texture and body of the cheese.

iii) The told salt is added in two-third portion of the milk an remaining third of milk is heated to 77°C (170 F) for 5-10 minutes and then mixed with the salted milk. The final temperature 40-60°C (105-115°F) thus achieved is suitable for renneting. It also improves the texture and body of the cheese and slightly reduces the total bacterial count.

For coagulation of milk about 22-23 ml. good quality rennet is required for 100 kg milk and it takes about 2-3 hours at 40-46°C temperature. The curd is ladled into metallic moulds or wooden frames and allowed to drain under adequate pressure to obtain a good firm cheese for easy handling. The pieces of fresh cheese are wrapped in cheese paper. Brine solution is usually prepared in whey available form the drainage of cheese. The cheese may be consumed fresh or ripened for 4-8 months in earthen pots.

The yield of Domiati cheese is dependent on the total solid content of milk and the concentration of salt added to milk (Table 4.20).

Table 4.20. Effect of salt quantity of the yield of domiati cheese

Kind of milk	Salt content in milk (%)				
	0	2.5	5.0	7.5	10.0
Buffalo milk	17.25	20.33	28.49	32.72	36.50
Cow milk	11.18	13.08	18.84	24.71	27.75

The average values of total solids, fat and salt are 45±4, 24±3 and 4.5±0.5 per cent in the fresh; and 48±0.6 per cent in the ripened.

2. **Provolone cheese:** Provolone cheese is prepared in Egypt particularly in the small dairies of Alexandria. It is usually prepared from the raw mixed milk fo cow and buffalo without addition of any starter. It is also prepared from raw milk of cow or buffalo. The raw milk is coagulated by adding a suitable quantity of rennet to obtain a good firm curd in one hour. The curd is cut and then allowed to remain in the whey for about 15

minutes. After this whey is drained out and the curd is transferred into a cloth lined metallic hoop and left for 2-3 hours.

The curd is now cut into small pieces and left at room temperature to make it more elastic. It can be tested by dipping a piece of curd in hot water bath at 79-80°C (175-176°F) for few seconds and then stretched slowly into a fine thread without the tendency to break. After this the curd pieces are dipped in hot water both at about 79-80°C to make more elastic, so that small balls may be prepared. The curd balls are then dipped into a 20 per cent salted whey solution s for 24 hours and then placed in a rope net hanging from ceiling for 24 hours smoking with the smoke burning woods in a half-cut barrel. The smoked cheese is then kept in ripening room at 10-12°C (50-54°F) for a period of 4 weeks and then used as a food item (El-Sokkary and Hassan 1952; El-Soda *et al.,* 197ga). The difference in chemical composition of milk and provolone cheese (Table 4.21) prepared from the raw whole milk of buffalo and cow is significant.

Table 4.21. Composition of milk and provolone cheese or buffalo (B) and cow (C) milk

Steps in cheese making	pH		Fat		Protein		Salt (%)	
	B	C	B	C	B	C	B	C
Whole milk	6.6	6.7	6.15	3.70	4.29	3.40	-	-
Curd before shaping	5.2	5.2	30.50	24.50	17.19	19.53	-	-
Cheese before salting	5.4	5.4	29.00	24.00	15.67	22.39	-	-
Salted cheese	5.3	5.3	30.35	25.50	18.34	22.40	2.68	2.20
Smoked cheese	5.4	5.3	32.50	28.00	21.87	-	2.74	2.64
Ripened cheese	5.5	5.4	36.50	30.00	20.25	24.10	3.12	2.98

Formation of adequate concentration of desired volatile fatty acids is important for the development of characteristic flavor in the cheese. Acetic acid is found during all the stage of provolone cheese making. Butyric acid appears during the early stages of cheese manufacture and propionic, caproic acid caprylic acids develop during the ripening period (El-Soda *et al.,* 1976b).

In raw milk of buffalo, bacterial, yeast and mould counts are usually high which significant decreases in cheese (Table 4.22). This is due to formation of lactic acid, heating during smoking and increase of acidity during ripening stages (El-Soda *et al.,* 1976c).

Table 4.22. Micorbial condition of milk and provolone cheese.

Microbial count	Raw buffalo milk	Provolone cheese
Total count x 10^6	0.0 -14.0	4.00-6.00
Lactic acid bacteria x 10^6	0.02-1.0	1.60-12.00
COliform bacteria x 10^3	10-1000	0.0
Enterococci x 10^3	2.30	0.0
Yeast and mould	Over count	0.0
Streptococcus faecalis	83.4	66.7
Str. Lactis/Str. Cremosis	16.6	22.9

3. **Mish cheese:** Mish is a popular cheese of Egypt. It has yellowish-brown colour, sharp flavor and high salt content. The exact origin of mish cheese is not known but supposed to be similar to salted cheese found in the Egyptian toms of king Hroaha of the first dynasty about 3200 BC (Iskander, 1942). It is popular dairy food of farmers and labourers of Egypt. Mish cheese can be prepared any time but large quantity is prepared during the winter season when large quantity of milk is available.

Mish cheese is prepared from karish cheese which is made of skim milk by lactic fermentation. Process of mish cheese manufacture differs from one to another region, but various steps are almost similar (hamdy and taha, 1954). The cubes of karish cheese are packed under microaerophilic conditions in a large clean earthen pot known as "ballas". The space between chyeese pieces are filled with whole milk, skim milk or butter milk containing about 10 per cent salt which is known as 'laban khad'. The other additives used are sesame oil cake (Kosba residue of ghee or Samma (Morta), oriental spices and medicinal plants and may be from 2-7 per cent of whole mixture. The ballas is covered by a palm leaf sheath and a piece of cloth and then tightly sealed with mud paste. The pores of ballas and mud seal keep the contents under partially anaerobic conditions during ripening period of about one year in a warm sunny place.

Thc moisture, fat, protein and salt content of mish cheese is about 55.76-74.14, 3.3 -18.0, 12.64-14. 16 and 10.3 -18.0 per cent in different samples. About 56.9, 81.1 per cent of the total nitrogen is present in the form of free amino nitrogen and arginine is almost absent (El-Erian *et al.,* 1975).

The ripened mish cheese is yellowish-brown in colour with a characteristic sharp, pungent flavor and somewhat butyric odour. The old ripen pickling medium of mish cheese is called mish paste which resembles with the cheese in chemical composition, flavor and odour (El-Gendy, 1983). The various volatile fatty acids present in the ripened mish cheese are acetic, propionic, butyric, caproic, caprylic and valeric acids and the characteristic odour is imparted byt eh alpha-keto butyric acid (Amin and El-Kholy, 1979).

4. **Shankalish cheese:** Shankalish is the native Syrian cheese almost similar to the mish cheese of Egypt (ABou-Donia and Abdel-Kader, 1979).

A coagulum of milk similar to karish cheese is prepared and collected in large containers. The curd is kneaded with 7.2 per cent powdered salt and a mixture of oriental spices according to taste and then shaped into balls of 3-4 cm diameter. The cheese is ripened in a dark humid-hot room till the development of a characteristic sharp flavor. The surfaces of ripened cheese is cleaned and the stored submerged in olive oil glass containers,or sun dried for 2-3 days for preventing the over ripening. The average moisture, protein, fat ash and salt content of shakalish cheese are 30.2, 46.6, 7.76, 7.02 and 5.5 per cent, respectively with mean pH value of 4.5. The cheese is free from enterobacteria and staphylococci but contain proteolitic, lypolytic and aerobic spore forming bacteria.

5. **Ricotta cheese:** Ricotta is a soft, fresh and unripened cheese of Italian origin, Ricotta cheese is prepared from the cheese whey in many Mediterranean and Scandinavian countries. Satisfactory ricotta cheese may be prepared from paneer whey. The paneer whey is first neutralized by mixing 1.0 per cent solution of calcium hydroxide. The paneer whey is first neutralized by mixing 1.0 per cent solution of calcium hydroxide. After this whyole milk and neutralized paneer whey are mixed in the ratio of 1:9 and then heated to 95°C. A dilute solution (1.0%) of citric acid is added slowly while stirring the mixture for coagulation. Heating is stopped and coagulum is left in the whey for 45-60 minutes and then strained through a muslin cloth applying gentle pressure for squeezing the whey. The soft ricotta cheese, thus obtained, is a rich source of protein, minerals and vitamin and consumed in different forms. Average yield of ricotta cheese is about 6 per cent from the peneer whey of buffalo milk (Shukla and Brar, 1986).

6. **Stracchino type cheese:** It is a soft cheese made from whole milk of buffalo. The technology of manufacture is quite simple (Mincione *et al.*, 1984) and can be adopted easily. Lots of 100 kg whole of buffalo milk iare filterd, standardized to 6 per cent fat by dilution with water or skimmed milk and pasteurized at 63°C for 30 per cent fat by dilution with water or skimmed milk and pasteurized at 63°C for 30 minutes. A lactic starter culture (commercial yoghurt in milk) is added at the rate of 1.2 per cent in the milk cooled to 43°C. After 10 minutes cultured milk is further cooled to 37°C for renneting (50 minutes total time). The curd is broken and separated from the whey and then cooled in moulds for about 5 hours, rrined for 2 hours in 20 per cent salt solution (4°SH) and then dried and ripened at 6°C and 80 per cent relative humidity for 21 days. The average yield of fresh cheese is about 23.6 per cent salt solution (4° SH) and then dried and ripened at 6°C and 80 per cent relative humidty for 21 days. The average yield of fresh cheese is about 23.6 per cent but final yield is only 16.1 percent due to approximately 31.5 per cetn loos during the ripening of cheese. The blocks of mature cheese of normally 14x 20 x 6 cm size had thin white to flesh colour skin, whitish coloour, compact and soft pasty mixture and delicate taste. It contains about 59 per cent fat, 5.4 per cent total nitrogen. 1.0-1.2 per cent titrable acidity (equivalent to lactic acid) and 1.7:1 ratio fo calcium:phosphorus on dry matter basis. Lactic acid bacteria count increases to maximum after about 14 days ripening and then declines. The ratio of lactobaccili to streptococci also increases to maximum 9:1 after 14 days but at the end of ripening period it is 1 to 1.5:1.

7. **Mozarella cheese:** It is a cheese made of fermented milk of high fat content. The cheese was developed in Italy and white Mozarella cheese made of buffalo milk is now spread worldwide. It is extensively used as spread in pizza making, which is also an Italian fast foods developed at Naples. The common four kinds of mozzarella cheese are standard mozzarella, low moisture mozzarella cheese, part skim mozzarella cheese and part skim low moisture mozzarella cheese (Table 4.23). Part skim mozzarella cheese demand is more due to low milk fat and high milk protein content. Increasing demand o mozzarella cheese in the global market has increased the farming of dairy type Indian buffaloes in many countries of almost all the countries.

Table. 4.23. Per cent composition of mozzarella cheese varieties

Sl	Variety	Moisture	Milk Fat	Mil Protein	Carbo-hydrates	Ash
1	Standard mozzarella cheese	52	22.5	20.5	2.0	3.0
2	Low moisture mozzarella cheese	45	24.5	22.0	2.5	3.0
3	Part Skim mozzarella cheese	52	16.5	25.5	3.0	3.0
4	Part Skim low moisture mozzarella cheese	45	17.0	25.0	3.0	3.3

Part skim mozzarella cheese is made from a mixture of three parts whole milk and one part skim milk of buffalo. The mixtures are standardized to contain minimum content of milk fat and maximum content of mixture (Table 4.24).

Table. 4.24. Standards of mozzarella cheese (%)

Sl.	Variety	Maximum moisture	Minimum milk fat
1	Standard mozzarella	52	20
2	Low moisture mozzarella	48	20
3	Part skim mozzarella	52	15
4	Part skim low moisture mozzarella	48	15

Cheese varieties contain most of the dietary essential minerals in the form of organic compounds and also vitamins (Table 4.25).

Table. 4.25. Minerals and vitamins in different mozzarella cheese (mg/100g).

Nutrients	Standard mozzarella	Low moisture Mozzarella	Part skim Mozzarella	Part skim low moisture Mozzarella
Minerals contents				
Calcium	528	575	6567	731
Magnesium 19.4	21	23.5	26	
Phosphorus	379	412	472	524
Potassium	68	75	86	95
Sodium	381	415	476	528

Trace Minerals				
Copper	0.02	0.022	0.026	0.027
Iron	0.18	0.20	0.22	0.25
Manganese	0.008	0.009	0.010	0.011
Selenium	0.0148	0.0161	0.1147	0.0163
Zinc	2.26	2.46	2.82	3.13
Fat soluble vitamins				
Vitamin A	0.246	0.274	0.181	0.191
Vitamin E	0.36	0.665	0.439	0.462
Water soluble vitamins				
B1 (Thiamin)	0.15	0.016	0.018	0.021
B2 (Riboflavin)	0.248	0.270	0.309	0.34
B6	0.057	0.062	0.071	0.079
B12	0.00066	0.00073	0.00084	0.00093
Folate	0.007	0.008	0.009	0.010
Niacin	0.086	0.094	0.107	0.119
Pantothenic acid	0.065	0.071	0.081	0.090
C (Ascorbic acid)	0	0	0	0

Cream

The high fat containing portion of milk obtained by either gravitational or mechanical concentration of whole milk is known as cream. According to the PFA rules (1976), cream should not contain less than 25 per cent milk fat.

Large variation occurs in the composition of cream. It is much richer in fat content than the milk and contains all the other milk constituents in lower proportion than in the whole milk. Cream may be classified into three types on the basis of fat percentage.

a) **Thin cream or light cream:** The cream containing less than 30 per cent butter fat is called thin or light cream. The cream obtained by gravity method is usually thin and contains 10-25 per cent fat milk. Thin cream may be also manufactured by centrifugal method for use in the preparation of coffee cerem, fruit cream and ice cream etc.

b) **Medium cream or whipping cream:** It is prepared by centrifugal method and contains 30-40 per cent milk fat. Market creams are normally medium type.

c) Rich/heavy/plastic cream: The cream containing more than 65 per cent milk fat is known as rich, heavy or plastic cream. It is rarely manufactured for marketing.

Cream is a high energy milk product and used as human food as follows:

i) Direct consumption of fresh and pasteurized cream in coffee and other foods.

ii) For the preparation of ice creams.

iii) For the preparation of sweet cream butter from fresh cream or sour/ripened cream butter from cultured cream or aged cream. The latter is manufactured by fermentation of cream with a known culture of milk fermenting microorganisms or natural dahi culture for the development of a characteristic aroma of ghee.

iv) For the manufacture of ghee either from sweet or ripened cream or the butter obtained from the churning of cream.

Composition of buffalo cream: The average chemical composition of different types of cream prepared from the whole milk of buffalo (Table 4.26) shows that various milk constituents separated in cream are negatively related with the percentage of milk fat.

Table 4.26. Composition of buffalo cream

Constituents (%)	Fat content in cream (%)			
	25	35	55	80
Total solids	32.6	41.5	59.5	82.0
Moisture	67.4	58.5	40.5	18.0
Solids not fat	7.6	6.5	4.5	5.0
Milk fat	25.0	35.0	550	30.0
Protein	3.1	2.6	1.8	0.8
Lactose	3.9	3.4	2.3	1.0
Ash	0.6	0.5	0.4	0.2

Butter

The compact milk fat concentrate obtained churning of sweet or ripened cream is known as butter. It may not contain salt and/or permitted colour.

According to PFA Rules (1976) butter should not contain less than 80 percent milk fat and more than 1.5 percent curd and colouring agents. Use of diacetyl as a flavor is permitted to maximum 4 ppm. Other additives for preservation like calcium hydroxide, sodium bicarbonate, sodium carbonate and sodium polyphosphate should not be more than 0.2 per cent. These characteristics are also applicable to makkhan obtained from the churning curd. Various types of butters normally available in the market are:

a) **Sweet cream butter:** Butter prepared from sweet cream or less than 0.2 per cent acidity.

b) **Salted sweet cream butter:** Butter obtained from sweet cream of less than 0.2 per cent acidity and containing about 3 per cent added common salt.

c) **Ripened cream butter:** Butter obtained from the churning of ripened cream. Normally dahi culture is used for the ripening of butter. Aging of cream to room temperature is also used for the development of a delicate butter aroma.

Fat globules of butter made from buffalo's milk cream are larger and butter contains about 68.56 per cent globular fat (Ismail and Sirry, 1966). Aging of buffalo cream for 12 hours at 10°C (50oF) helps in satisfactory crystallization of the fat (Nabar *et al.,*., 1969). Butter is a popular dairy product in human dietary and used as follows:

a) Direct consumption: Normally fresh or pasteurized butter is used as table butter for eating with bread, chapatti, dal and rice etc.

b) Manufacture of ghee: Butter obtained from ripened cream is preferably used for the preparation of ghee of pleasant characteristic aromas.

c) Used as a cooking medium

d) Used for the preparation of sweets like butter soma.

Butter Oil

Clarified milk fat obtained after the removal of moisture and solids not fat from the cream or butter is known as butter oil. It is known as dry milk fat, dehydrated butter fat or anhydrous milk fat. This similar to ghee of India and somna of Egypt.

Butter oil contains about 99.5 -99.8 per cent milk fat and traces of moisture acidity is normally below 0.5 per cent and peroxide value is less than 0.1 per cent.

Butter oil is used as a cooking medium, preparation of sweets and reconstituted milk after mixing with skimmed milk powder and water.

Ice Cream

Ice cream is a frozen dairy product prepared from the mixture of sweet cream and common sugar (sucrose). It may not contain permissible flavor, colour and stabilizer.

According to the PFA Rules (1976) of India, ice cream should not contain less than 10 per cent milk fat, 3.5 per cent milk protein and 36 per cent total milk solids. The concentration of permitted stabilizers and emulsifiers must not exceed 0.5 per cent. Special ice cream may be prepared by the addition of one or more edible additives like fruits, fruit juice, eggs, nuts, dry fruits and chocolate. These products must not contain less thatn 8 per cent milk fat. Starch may be added upto 5 per cent and must be declared prominently on the container of ice cream. Ice cream premix standard composition of ice cream fixed by the Indian Standards Institution vide its resolution number IS:2802 of 1964 is given in (Table 4.27).

Table 4.27. ISI Specification of ice cream

Constituents	Content
Minimum weight , g/litre	525
Total solids (%) Min.	36.0
Minimum milk fat (%)	10.0
Maximum acidity as lactic acid (%)	0.25
Maximum stabilizers/ emulsifiers (%)	0.5
Standard plate count per g	<2,50,000
Coliform bacteria per g	<90
Phosphatase test	Negative

Various types of ice creams are prepared in different countries but there appears to be no standard classification of ice cream for the international acceptance. Flavoured ice cream, chocolate ice cream, fruits cream or phaluda, nut cream and soft ice cream (Softy) are quite popular in different countries. Demand of softy is more than the other kinds of ice creams and children are very fond of eating softy. It contains about 3-6 per cent milk fat, 11-14 per cent other milk solids, 12-15 per cent added sugar, 0.4-0.5 per cent stabilizers and emulsifiers and permitted flavor and colour. Softy is drawn at about -8°C (18°F) and served for eating in cones of starch and gelatin molded in attractive shapes.

Good quality ice cream should be palatable and soft and it should not be rancid, bitter, coarse and sandy. Ice cream is generally eaten a frozen dessert, while softy is taken during lunch break and pleasure trips to market, parts, cinema circus and other places of recreation and relaxation.

Indian Milk Products

The nutritional contribution of milk of buffalo and other farm animals was recognized in ancient India thousands of years ago. The various milk products developed in the Indian subcontinent are referred as Indian milk products. Due to high fat and total milk solids percentage most of the Indian dairy products are preferably prepared form the buffalo milk. Dahi, ghee and paneer are most common dairy products of Indian sub-continent. Chhanna and khoa or mawa are coagulated and concentrated milk products, respectively, which are the base of a large variety of sweets prepared in the Indian sub-continent. The common dairy products of India may be identified into the following three broad groups:

1. Concentrated whole milk products like kheer/ basundi/ tasmai/ havya, khoa or mawa, rabbri, kulfi
2. Coagulated milk products are paneer and chhana
3. Cultured milk products are dahi and srikhand or chakka.
4. Products of concentrated butter fat industry are cream, makkhan, ghee lassi and ghee residue.

Kheer: Kheer is prepared by the partial dehydration of whole milk in a pan by direct heating. Usually small quantity of rice and occasionally dry fruits and nuts are added and boiled to cook. Sufficient quantity of sugar is added in the last stage of boiling. Kheer prepared from milk standardized to 4 per cent fat content and containing 2.5 per cent washed rice and 5 per cent sugar may contain about 67 per cent moisture, 7.83 per cent fat, 6.34 per cent protein, 8.45 per cent lactose, 1.41 per cent ash and 8.95 percent added sugar (De *et al.*, 1976).

Rabri: A concentrate and sweetened whole milk product containing scattered clotted cream is known as rabri. Sugar is added at the rate of 5-6 per cent of the original volume of milk. Rabri is normally prepared by direct heating of milk in a shallow pan. The approximate content of moisture. Ft. protein added sugar, lactose and ash in rabri is 30, 20, 10, 20, 17 an 3 per cent, respectively (Singh *et al.*, 1975).

Khurchan: Khurchan is prepared by simmering whole milk without stirring in a shallow pan on direct fire. This helps in slow evaporation of moisture. Finely powdered sugar is normally mixed at the time of eating. It contains about 27.9, 23.6, 15.4, 14.9, 15.2 and 3.0 per cent moisture, milk fat, protein, lactose, added sugar and ash, respectively (Gupta and Rao, 1972).

Malai or Sarhi or Sar: The upper layer of fat rich elastic layer (milk skin) removed from the boiled milk after cooling slowly at room temperature is called malai. It is available normally in home and also at eh halwai-shop. Drinking milk sellers of Indian sub-continent invariably put a small piece of malai at the top milk. Malai is also referred to the skin of curd and served at the top of sweet lassi commonly sold in summer.

Kulfi: It is a concentrated, sweetened, flavoured and frozen milk product. It may also contain pieces of dry fruits and nuts. The product is frozen in different shapes to make it more attractive. Its composition is variable. Good quality kulfi may be prepared from mixed cow and buffalo milk concentrated to contain about 26 per cent total solids (Salooja, 1979).

Khoa or Mawa: The partially dehydrated whole milk prepared by direct heating in a pan is known as khoa or mawa the milk is constantly stirred and scrapped from the sides of pan with the help of a khunti while heating till it becomes semi-solid. After this content is cooled at room temperature and made in different shapes for marketing. It should not contain less than 20 per cent milk fat (IS:4883, 1968).

The chemical composition of khoa depends on the composition of raw milk and khoa prepared from buffalo milk may contain about 91.2, 37.1, 17.8, 22.1 and 3.6 per cent moisture, milk fat, protein, lactose and ash, respectively (Ray and De, 1952). Khoa of uffalo milk is dull white, soft, slightly greasy and rich. Its texture may be smooth or grandular. Khoa is base material for the preparation of famous sweets like peda, burfi, gulab Jamun, kalajamun, kalakand, ghujia *etc.*

Paneer: It is prepared by the rennet coagulation of whole milk. It is an indigenous soft cheese of India. The different varieties of paneer are surati, bandal and dacca. Average yield of surati paneer of buffalo milk is 34 per cent. The moisture, total solids and fat contents in surati paneer are 71.1, 28.9 and 11.1 per cent, respectively (Bhattacharya *et al.*, 1971). Good quality paneer is prepared by coagulating the milk at about 80°C at pH 5 (Vishweshwaraish, 1979).

Chhanna: CHhanna is prepared by the coagulation of boiled hot whole milk with lactic acid, lemon juice or chhanna whey. According to PFA Rules (1976) it should contain more than 70 per cent moisture. The fat content should not be less than 50 per cent of dry matter in chhanna. Average values of moisture, fat, protein,lactose and ash in chhanna of buffalo milk are 51.6, 29.6, 14.4, 2.3 and 2.0 per cent, respectively (Ray and De, 1953). Good quality chhana may be prepared by coagulationg whole milk with citric acid at 70°C (Kundu and De, 1972; Iyer, 1978; Ahmed *et al.*, 1981).

In the process of chhanna making the heating of milk favours greater recovery of milk protein but loss of soluble nutrients remains unaffected (Table 4.28). A higher loss of fat occurs in the manufacture of chhanna from buffalo milk (Ray and De, 1953). The yield of chhanna from buffalo milk is 22 to 24 per cent of which about 50 per cent is moisture. Homogenization of milk before coagulation results in higher yield due to more recovery of milk solids without affecting of the quality of chhanna (jagtap and Shukla, 1973). The chhanna of buffalo milk is whitish, slightly hard, coarse and greasy. Chhanna may be stored for several days at refrigeration temperature but not more than 2 days at the room temperature.

Table 4.28. Distribution of milk constituents in chhanna and chhanna-whey of buffalo milk (%).

Milk constituents	Chhanna	Chhanna-whey
Total milk solids	65	35
Solids not fat	48	52
Milk fat	85	15
Mil protein	91	9
Lactose	12	88
Total ash	60	40

Good quality sweet chhanna is extensively used for the preparation of the famous Bengali sweets like rasgulla, pantoa, khirmohan, cham-cham and khurma etc.

Dahi: Dahi or curd is a coagulated milk product obtained from boiled or pasteurized milk by acid fermentation with the help of natural lactic acid bacteria or specific harmless bacterial culture. Normally diluted curd is used as culture which is also known as starter or jaman.

Dahi may be prepared from whole as well as skim milk. The former is an intermediary step in the manufacture of makhan and ghee. Dahi may be classified into the following three types:

i) **Sweet or midly sour dahi:** It is slightly acidic and lactic acid content (acidity) does not exceed 0.7 per cent by weight. A mixed culture of Streptococcus lactis. Str. Diacetilactics and Snd Sir cremoris is used for the curdling of milk. Dahi is sweet or mildly sour with a pleasant characteristic aroma.

ii) **Sour dahi:** It has sharp acidic flavor. Starter for sour dahi preparation contains Lactobacillus bulgaricus or Str. Thermophillus or both in addition to those responsible for the curdling of sweet dahi. The acidity as lactic acid should not be more thatn 1.0 per cent by weight.

Both type of dahi should be negative for phosphatase test and should not contain more than 100 cells of yeast and mould and 10 cells of coliform bacteria pper gram of dahi. The milk solids in dahi are normally 5-10 per cent higher than the original milk. Dahi prepared from whole milk of buffalo contains 6-8 per cent milk, fat, 18-20 per cetn total solids and 0.8-1.0 per cent acidity. In dahi of boiled milk about half of the total fat is present in one per cent top layer and less thatn 8 per cent in the bottom layer. The difference may be still greater in a dahi of raw milk (Anantakrishnan and Kothavalla, 1946). Stirring of milk after 2-4 hours of inoculation with starter improves the uniformity of fat globules in dahi (Devengan *et al.*, 1970). Use of higher level of starter (2.5 per cent) produces more firm dahi than the low level and uneven distribution of fat globules is also reduced (Oommen, 1972).

Dahi has been found to better milk food for lactose intolerant infants (Chandrasekaran *et al.*, 1975). Buffalo milk dahi is a richer source of available nutrients thatn the cow's milk dahi (Khambatta and dastur, 195). Dahi eating helps in the prevention of putrefactive processes and corrects various digestive disorders.

Sweetened dahi/Lal dahi/ Payodhi: This kind of dahi is prepared in the eastern part of India. Payodhi has a characteristic brown colour, cooked flavor and firm texture. It contains 6-7 per cent added sugar preferably before boiling. Sweetened dahi is normally set in earthenware known as nadi or kahantari and takes about 15-16 hours for proper setting (Ray and Srinivasan, 1972).

Chakka: The solid mass obtained from the partial straining of whole milk dahi through a muslin or cheese cloth is known as chakka. The composition of chakka is quite variable (Table 4.29) and depends on the composition of milk, degree of lactic fermentation and drainkage of whey (Date of Mahajan, 1971). Chakka is the basic ingredient for the preparation of Srikhand and also prepared for easy transportation to long distance.

Table 4.29. Composition of chakka (%)

Samples	Moisture	Fat	Protein	Ash	Lactic acid
1	63.2	14.7	-	-	0.80
2	59.6	22.4	10.3	1.03	2.32

Srikhand: Srikhand is a sweetened dairy product, prepared from the whey strained curd known as chakka. Chakka is throughtly mixed with 30-50 pr cent powdered sugar. Flavouring agents and colour like saffaron 20 ml. of 0.6 per cent solution, 2g nutmeg powder and 1.5 -2.0 g cardamom seeds are generally mixed in a 1 kg chakka (Ingle and Joglekar, 1974). An acceptable srikhand may contain 60 percent total solids, 42 per cent sugars and 7 per cent protein (Aneja *et al.*, 1978). Srikhand is a popular dairy product of Gujarat, Maharashtra and Karnataka in India. It is also used for the preparation of srikhandgolla. A dough prepared from chakka, maize flour and baking powder is made into small balls and fried in boiling ghee or edible oil and then soaked in sugar syrup for the preparation of srikhandgola (Waghmare, 1977). Srikhand and srikhand products have a short shelf slife at room temperature in tropical climatic conditions. Incorporation of antioxidants, dehydration to less than 9 per cent moisture content and storage below 10°C at a dry place may significantly increase the keeping quality and products may be stored for 4-6 weeks period without significant changein the taste.

Makkhan: A concentrate milk fat product similar to butter and obtained from the curning of whoel milk dahi by indigenous method is known as makkhan or navneer or layanu. According to the PFA rules (1976) it should not contain less thatn 76 per cent milk fat. On an average makkahn contains 18-20 per cent moisture. 76-80 per cent butter fat. 1-1.5 per cent non fat milk solids and acidity normally does not exceed 0.2 per cent makkhan obtained from buffalo milk is light greenish-white in colour, hard and granular with a pleasant and slightly acid aroma when fresh. The recovery of makkhan is almost equal to fat percentage int eh initial milk because the minor loss of fat in lassi or mattha is compensated for by the overrun in the makkhan.

Keeping quality of mkkhan is relatively low and normally processed for ghee making after 7-10 days colletion, keeping quality may be significantly improved by storing the makkhan in butter milk which should be changed daily. It is further improved by storage in 0.8 per cent lactic acid solution (Rangappa and Banerjee, 1948).

Fresh makkhan is used for direct consumption with cooked foods in the Indian subcontinent. Large quantity of makkhan is converted into ghee and a small amount is sometimes used for the preparation of indigenous tonics with other medicinal ingredients.

Ghee-clarified butter fat: Ghee or clarified butter fat is a rich source of energy and produced by dehydration of makkhan, butter or cream by cooking at 110-120°C. Ghee has been used as ain important food item since the vedic period in the Indian sub-continent (Yegna Narayana Aiyer, 1953). It is also a popular dairy product of the Arabic countires and common known as samna (El-Sokkary and Zaki, 1956).

Ghee is prepared by the following three methods viz. desi method, creamery-butter method and direct cream method. Recovery of fat is significantly affected by the method of ghee preparation (Table 4.30) due to loss of fat in different fractions of processing (Misra and Kushwaha, 1970). Higher fat recovery is possible from the high fat and washed creams (De and Srinivasan, 1958; Madan Pal and Rajoria, 1975). Similarly recovery of ghee from makkhan in desi method can be significantly increased by the use of improved technique of dahi churning (Jain *et al.*, 1947).

Table 4.30. Average milk fat recovery of ghee by different methods.

Method	Loss of fat (%)				Fat recovery (%)
	Skim milk	Lassi/ buttern milk	Ghee residue	Handling	
Desi method	-	13.2	1.9	2.5	82.4
Creamery butter	1.4	0.8	1.4	4.5	91.6
Direct cream	1.4	-	9.0	1.7	87.7

Average composition of buffalo ghee is as follows:

Fat percentage	:	99-99.5
Moisture content	:	not more than 0.5%
Carotene content	:	Traces
Vitamin A activity	:	17-38μ per g of fat
Tocopherol	:	18-37μ per g of fat
Free fatty acids	:	maximum 2.8%

Physical qualities of ghee: The colour of ghee is affected by the method of preparation and buffalo ghee is white with a greenish tinge when prepared by desi and creamery-butter methods but waxy-white on preparation by direct cream method (Lalitha and Dastur, 1956).

A pleasant, cooked and rich flavoured ghee of mildly sour acidity is preferred over the characteristic flat flavor of fresh milk fat.

Large grains of uniform size are desired in good quality market ghee.

Good quality ghee should not be smoky and over cooked or undercooked. Rancidity, greasiness, burnt colour and high sediments are unwanted characteristics of ghee and reduce its market value.

The problem of adulteration of desi ghee with other fats and oils is frequently encountered. The common adulterants of ghee are:

a) Hydrogenated vegetable oils

b) Refined vegetable oils

c) Animal body fat like tallow and lard.

Sometimes small qnatity of rice, smashed potato and banana are mixed in the adulterated ghee for improving the consistency.

Uses of ghee

i) Direct consumption with chapatti, cooked pulse soup and vegetable curry etc.

ii) Medium for cooking and frying and

iii) In confectionary

Lassi/chhanchh/mattha: The residual dahi left after the removal of makkhan by curing is known as lassi, channchh or mattha in different parts of the Indian sub-continent. Approximately 50-55 kg lassi is obtained for each kg of ghee production. The compositoni of mattha varies significantly and it depends on the rate of dilution during churning of dahi or the removal of makkhan. It contains about 90-96 per cent water, 4-10 per cent total solids and 0.4-0.6 per cent lactic acid.

Uses of Lassi

i) Direct consumption as a beverage, sugar, salt and spice, ice and flavor are used according to the taste and availability.

ii) As starter for the setting of dahi by indigenous method.

iii) For the preparation of curry and dahiwala etc.

Ghee residue: The semi-solid cooked residue obtained after the removal of ghee is called ghee residue. It may be light to dark brown in colour and contains 33-80 per cent milk fat. Large variation occurs in the chemical composition of ghee residue (Table 4.31) obtained by different methods of ghee making (Prahlad, 1954).

Table 4.31. Average compositon of buffalo ghee residue

Method of ghee making	Percent content				
	Water	Fat	Protein	Lactose	Ash
Desi method	13.4	33.4	32.8	15.4	5.2
Creamery butter	5.7	65.0	25.5	Traces	3.8
Unwashed cream	4.1	63.2	18.0	12.3	2.4
Washed cream	17	80.8	16.2	Traces	1.3

Uses: It is normally used for consumption mixed with sugar and may be also used for the preparation of sweets and milk toffees.

References

Abd-El-Salam, M.H. and El-Shibiny, S. 1966. The chemical composition of buffalo milk. I Genral composition. Indian J. Dairy Sci., 19:151-154.

Abu-Donia, Y.I. and Abdel-Hader, Y.I. 1979. Microbial flora and chemical composition of native Syrian hard cheese 'Mesanarah', "Medaffarah' and 'Shankalish'. Egyptian J. Dairy Sci., 7:211-229 (Fide Dairy Sci., abst., 42:3788).

Ahmed, A.R., Vyas, S.H., Upadhaya, K.G> and Thakkar, P.N. 1981. Study on manufacture of chhanna from buffalo milk. Gujarat Agric. Univ. Res. J., 7:32-36.

Ahuja, S.P., Shkhija, P.S. and Bhatia, I.S. 1972. Utilisation of fat by milch bufflaoes (*Bos bubalus*): the effect of amount of type of dietary lipids on milk fat secretion in lactating buffaloes. Indian J. Anim. Sci., 42: 167-173.

Akhundov, D. 1958. Chemcial composition of milk of Azerbaijan buffaloes. Sots. S-Kh., Azarb., 3:19-21 (fide Dairy Sci., Abst. 22:1708).

Adhundov, K.R. 1966. Changes in the compositon of buffalo's milk depending upon the season and calving period. Trudy. Azerb. Nanchno. Issled. Vet. Inst. 20:238-244 (fide Dairy Sci., Abst. 30: 321 & 2505).

Alim, K.A. 1975. A report on general aspects of studies on animal production buffalo and cattle in the Philippines. World Rev., Anim. Prod. 11:69-70.

Alim, K.A., Barbari, A. and Badram, A. 1977. Management trials on milking technique and concentrate feeding with local cattle and buffalo.World Rev. Anim. Prod., 13:27-32.

Alasafar, T. and Juma, K.H. 1970. Studies on Iraqui buffalo milk with reference to the effect of month of lactation. II. Compositon and some properties.Tropic. Agric., Trinidad, 47: 175-179.

Anantakrishnan, C.P. anmd Kothavalla, Z.R. 1946. Distribution for fat in dahi. Indian J. Vet Sci. Anim. Husb., 16:56-64.

Aneja, R.P., Vyas, M.N. , Thareja, V.K. and Nanda, K. 1978. Development of an industrial process for the manufacture of Srikhand. Proc. Inter. Dairy cong., New Delhi. Pp. 992.

Asker, A.A., Bedeir, L.H. and Kamal, T.H. 1957. The effect of stage of lactation on the composition of the buffalo milk and correlation between milk constituents. Indian J. Dairy Sci., 10:204-212.

Asker, A.A., Bedeir, LH., El-Itriby, A.A., Ahmed, I/A. and Khishin, S.S. 1971. Factors affecting butter fat content in Egyptian buffaloes. Anim. Prod. UAR, 9:181-187.

Basu, K.P., Paul, T.M., Shroff, H.B. and Rahman, M.A. 1948. Composition of milk and ghee. Final report of the scheme. Report series No. 8, ICAR, New Delhi.

Basu, S.B., Sarma, P.A., Nagarcenkar, R. and Sadana, D.K. 1979. Buffalo breeding studies on butter fat and SNF percentage. Annual Report. NDRI, Karnal. Pp. 177-178.

Bhargava, R.K. and Murdia, C.K. 1980. Research project report (1978-80). All Indian coordinated Research project on Buffaloes. Vallabhanagar, Udaipur.

Bhattacharya, D.C., Mathour, O.N., Srivasa, M.R. and Samlik, O 1971. Sutdies on the method of production and shelf life of peneer (cooking type of acid coagulated cottage cheese). J. Fd. Sci. Technol., 8: 117-120.

Bhimasena Rao, M. and Dastur, N.N. 1955. Hydrogen ion concentration of milk. 1. pH of milk of animal fo different breeds and individuals. Indian J. Dairy Sci., 8: 158-172.

Chandrasekaran, R., Kumar, V., Walia, B.N.S. and Moorthy, B. 1975. Carbohydrate intolerance in infants with acute diarrhea and its complication. Acta Paediatrica Scandinavica, 64:483-488.

Dalay, B.K., Abd-El-Mottaleb, L., El-Shazly, A. and Abdallah, R. 1976. The copoposition of buffaloes in mosul area. Mesopotamia j.Agric 11:55-60 (fide Dairy Sci) Abst., 39:67-90.

Dass, P.C. and Basu, S.B. 1975. Diurnal variation milk secretion of Murrah buffaloes, Indian j. Dairy Sci. 28:135-136.

Dass, P.C., Basu, S.B. and Sharma, K.N.S. 1976. Effect of frequency of milking on Murrah buffaloes. Indian J.Dairy Sci.29:113.-116.

Date, W.B. and Bhatia, D.S> 1955. Preservation of Indian milk sweets: Some preliminary studies on Srikhand wadi and milk burfee. Indian J. Diary Sci. 8:61-66.

De, S. and Srinivasan, M.R. 1958. Prodution and marketing of ghee. I. Production. Indian Dairyman, 10:156-160 & 165.

De, S. Thompkinson, D.K. Gahlot, D.P.a dn Mathur, O.N. 1976. Studies on methods of preparation and preservation of kheer. Indian J. Dairy Sci., 29: 316-318.

Devangan, M.L., Ogra, J.L. and Rao, Y.S. 1970. Studies on fat globules, Balwant Vidyapeeth J. Agric., Sci. Res., 10:19-22.

Dilanyan, Z., Agababyan, I.A. and Aslanayan, E. 1971. Characteristics of protein in buffaloes milk and some products made from it. Proc., Intern. Uni. Dairy Conf. Baku, pp. 359-263 (Fide Dairy Sci., Ast. 34:1856).

Dzafarov, T.A. 1969. The effect of age (in calvings) on content of protein, fat and dry matter in buffalo milk. Uchen. Zap. Azab., Sel'-Khoz. Inst. Ser. Zhivot. 1:94-96 (fide Dairy Sci., Abst., 39:1544).

El_erian, A.F.M., Farag, a.H. and El-Gindy, S.M. 1975. Chemical studies on mish cheese. Agric. Res. Rev. UAR. 53:173-181.

El-Ghandour, M.A., El-Gazzar, H. and Youniss, N.A. 1979. Studies on the buffalo's and cow's milk in the upper in the upper part of Egypt. Res. Bull. Faculty Agric., Alin Sharma Univ., 977-979 (fide Dairy Sci. Abst., 41:6294-96).

El-Soda, M.A., El-Hagarawy, I.S., Rakshy, S.E.S.E. and Abou-Donia, S.A. 1976b. Studies on provolone cheese. II. Changes in the volatile fatty acids during processing and ripening Indian J. Dairy Sci., 29:355-358.

El-Shazly, A., Sharara, H.A. and Fahmi, A.H. 1974. Some factors affecting physical and chemical properties of Egyptian cow's and buffalo's milk. 3. Variations due to different milking portions. Milchwissenchaft, 29: 355-358.

El-Sokkary, A.H. and Hassan, H.A. 1952. Lactose and chloride content of Egyptian cows and buffaloes milk. Analyst., 75: 143-146 (fide Dairy Sci. Abst., 12:191).

El-Sokkary, A.H. and Zaki, M.H. 1956. Effect of stage of lactation and individuality of animal on the stability of resultant samna. Anim. Agric. Sci., Cairo, 1(1): 83-105 (fide Anim. Breed Abst., 27:675).

Fahmy, A.H. and Sharara, H.A. 1950. Studies on Egyptian Domiati cheese. J. Dairy Res., 17:312-328.

Fahmy, A.H., Sharara, H.A. and El-Shazly, A. 1974. Some factors affecting physical and chemical properties of Egyptian cows and buffalo's milk Mitchwissenchaft, 29: 599-601.

Ganguly, S., BOman, T.J., Dastur, N.N. and Vaccha, S.M. 1959. Chemical composition of chakka. Indian J. Dairy Sci., 12:121-124.

Ghosh, S.N. and Ananta Krishnan, C.P. 1963. Compositoin of milk. IV. Infuence of seson, breed and species. Indian J. Dairy Sci., 17: 190-192.

Gotsiridze, N. and Kitoshvili, I. 1981. The effectiveness of buffalo breeding. Zhivotnovodstov, 3:37-38 (fide Anim. Breed. Abst., 49-5687).

Grigorov, H.Y.l, Shalichev, Ye and Goranov, N. 1962. Composition and properties of buffalo's milk. Proc. XVII Imer. Dairy Cong. A. 209.

Gupta, M.P.a dn Rao, Y.S. 1972. Chemcial quality of khurchan. Indian J. Dairy Sci. 25:70-72.

Hamdy, M.K. and Taha, S.M. 1954. Mish: A soft ripened Egyptain cheese. Milk Prod. J., 45 (11): 14-15 & 29-33. (fide Dairy Sci., Abst. 17:116).

Hanna, A.K., Hassan, A., Yassen, A. and Badawy, a. 1979. The effectiveness of subcutaneously versus intramuscular administration of oxytocin upon removal of residual milk in buffaloes and cattle. Alexandria J. Agric. Res., 27:567-574. (fide Dairy Sci., Abst. 42:6554).

Ingle, U.M. and Jogickar, N.V. 1974. Effect of fat and sugar variation on the acceptability of Srikhand preparations. J. Food Sci., Technol: India, 11:189, 190.

Ishaq, S.M. and Shah, S.K. 1975. Comparative performance of buffaloes and Sahiwal cows as dairy animals. Agric. Pakistan, 26:75-88 (fide Diary Sci., Abst. 41:569).

Ismail, A.A. and Sirry, I. 1966. Technological aspets of butter made from cows and buffalo milk. Alexandria J. Agric. Res., 13: 161-173 (fide Dairy Sci. 1bst., 29:2604).

Iyer, M. 1978. Physico-chemical studies on chhanna from cow's and buffalo's milk. M.Sc., Thesis, Kurukshetra University, Kurukshetra.

Jagtap, G.E. and Shulka, P.K. 1973. A note on the factors affecting the yield and quality of chhanna. J. Food Sci. Technol., 10:73-74.

Jain, D.H., Srinivasan, M.R. and Desai, K.K. 1947. Studies on the curd process of ghee manufacture. Rural India, 10: 201-205.

Kapoor, M. and Ludri, R.S. 1984. Effect of different milking intervals in buffaloes on secretion rates of milk and some of its organic constituents. Indian J. Anim. Sci. 54:153-157.

Khambatta, J.S. and Dastur, N.N. 1950. Nutritive value of dahi - rat feeding epermients. Indian J. Dairy Sci., 3:87-93.

Khan, M.A., Choudhary, M.Z, Qureshi, M.J. and Dar, Z.I. 1970. Influence of season on butter fat and protein coment in buffalo milk W. Pakistan J. Agric. Res., 8: 313-317.

Kulkarni, P.S. and Dole, K.K. 1956. Investigations in viscosity of milk. Indian J. Dairy Sci., 9: 68-79.

Kumar, A. and Tripathi, V.N. 1978. Effects of levels and methods of pre-partum and post-partum feeding on the yield and composition of milk and cost of milk production in Murrah buffaloes. Haryana Agric. Univ. J. Res., 8: 125-129.

Kumar, A., Singh, L.N., yadav, P.L. and Pandey, H.S. 1980. Studies on buffalo mok constituents during complete lactation. Fincal Project Report, IVRI, Izatnagar.

Kundu, S.S. and De, S. 1972. Chhanna producton from buffalo milk. Indian J. Dairy Sci. 25:159-163.

Lalitha, K.R. and Dastur, N.N. 1956. Colour development in desi ghee. Indian J. Dairy Sci., 9: 143-893.

Madan, Pal and Rajoria, G.S. 1972. Effect of multiple separation of cream on phospholipid content in ghee. Indian J. Anim. Res. 6:4-8.

Mahajan, B.M. 1971. Studies on the production and shelf life of spray dried srikhand. M.Sc. Thesis, Punjab University, Chandigarh.

Merzametov, M.M. 1965. Buffalo milk a valuable food. VOP. Pitan, 24: 76-78 (fide Dairy Sci. Abst., 27: 3617).

Minmeri, L., Franciscis, G. De and Interiefi, F. 1965. Relationship between pH, acidity and composition of buffalo milk. Acta Med. Vet. Nepali, 11:107-114 (fide Dairy Sci. Abst., 28:1676).

Minieri, L., Interieri, F. and Pane, G. 1967.Effect of lactation number on milk yield and composiotn in buffaloes. Acta Med. Vet. Nepali, 13:251-261 (fide Dairy Sci. Abst., 30:1053).

Mishra, R.C.a dn Kushwaha, N.S. 1970. Studies on methods of preparation of ghee. Indian J. Dairy Sci., 23:115-117.

Nabar, A.B., Srinivasan, M.R. and Iya, K.K. 1969. Studies on the water insoluble acids of cream and butter from buffalo milk. Indian J. Dairy Sci., 22:121-127.

Olenov, Yu, M. 1954. Causes for the differences beteen the butterfat content of portions of milk obtained after milk. Dokl. Akad. Nauk., SSSR, 97(2):361-364 (fide Dairy Sci. ABst., 17:230).

Oommen, S. 1972. The distribution of ft and fat globules in dahi. Indian J. Dairy Sci., 25:184-188.

Pandey, H.S. 1981. Genetic studies on the milk constituents of buffalo and their association with rlated traits. Ph.D. Thesis, Rohilkhand University, Bareilly.

Parekh, H.K.B. and Gangwar, P.C. 1968. Chemical composition of buffalo milk. Indian J. Dairy Sci., 21:171-182.

Patel, B.M., Dharni, B.M. and Patel, C.A. 1969. Studies on the effect of partial green feeding over dry feeding to milch bufflaoe. Indian J. Dairy Sci., 22:17-20.

Polikhronov, D. and Tosev, A. 1970. Functional characters of udder quarters in local buffaloe. Zhivot. Nauk., 7(3): 11-15 (fide Anim. Breed. ABst. 40:205).

Polikhronov, D. Bolkovski, S. and Peeva, T.S. 1978. Some lactation characters in Murrah and Bulgarian buffaloes and their F.1 corsses. Zhivot Nauk., 14:25-29 (fide Dairy Sci., Abst., 40: 3224).

Rangappa, K.S. and Banerjee, B.N. 1948. Storage of indigenous butter. Indian J. Dairy Sci., 1 : 45-47.

Raghab, M.T., Asker, A.A. and Kamal, T.H. 1958. The effect of age and season of calving on composiotn of Egyptian buffalo milk. Indian J. dairy Sci., 11:18-28.

Rao, M.K. and Nagarcenkar, R. 1977. Potentialities of the bufflo. World Rev. Anim. Prod. 13(3):53-62.

Ray, H.P. and Srinivasan, R.A. 1972. Use of microorganisms for producton of indigenous fermented milk products (sweetened dahi). Fd. Sci. technol. 9:62-65.

Ray, S.C. and De, S. 1952. Indigenous milk products of India. II. Khoa. Indian Dairy Men, 4:27-29.

Ray, S.C. and De, S. 1952. Indigenous milk products of India. III. Chhanna. Indian Dairy Mean, 5:14-17.

Salerno, A. 1967. Cited by H.S. Pandey in Ph.D. Thesis. Rohilkhand University, Bareilly.

Salooja, M.K. 1979. Studes on standardization on techniques for kulfi production M.Sc. Thesis. Kurukshetra University, Kurukshetra.

Schneder, B.H., Warner, J.N., Dharni, I.D., Agarwal, B.P., Sukhatme, P.V., Pendarkar, V.G. and Shankaran, A.N. 1948. The composiotn of milk. Misc. Bull. 61, ICAR, New Delhi.

Shalichev, Ye and Polikhronov., D. 1969. Composition and properties of milk of Murrah Buffaloes imported from India. Zhivot. Nauki, Sofia, 6:57-62 (fide Dairy Sci. Abst., 33:3135).

Shatichev, Ye, Tanev, G. and Polikhronov, D. 1975. Milk yield and compositon of purebred Murrah buffaloes and their crosses with Bulgarian buffloes. Zhivot. Nauki, Sofia, 12:73-77 (fide Dairy Sci. Abst., 38:3976).

Sharma, U.P., Rao, S.K. and Zariwala, I.T. 1980. Composition of milk of different breeds of buffaloes. Indian J. Dairy Sci., 33:7-12.

Shukla, K.S., Ranjhan, S.K. and Netke, S.P. 1972. Effect of various rates of concentrate feeding on the efficiency of milk producton in Murrah buffaloes. Indian J. Anim. Prod., 3:37-64.

Soni, P.L., Gangwar, P.C., Bagha, C.S., Srivastava, R.K. and Dhingra, D.P. 1980. Effect of environmental cooling on milk yield and certain milk constituents in buffaloes. Indian J. Nutr. Dietet. 17:220-227.

Singh, R.P., Singh, M., Rao, Y.S. and Singh, S.N. 1961. Quantitative relations amont the milk constituents. 1. Effect of breed, stage of lactation and age of animals. Indian J. Dairy Sci. 14:119-129.

Singh, R., Ogra, J.L. and Rao, Y.S. 1975. Observations on the microbial quality of some indigenous concentrated milk products. Indian J. Dairy Sci., 28:304-305.

Stewart, A.D. and Banerjee, 1930-31. Indian J. Med. Res., 18:57.

Tiwana, M.S., Bhullar, M.S. and Bhalaru, S.S., 1980. Indian Coordinated Research Project on Buffalo Breeding. Progress Report of Ludhiana Centre. 5th workshop. University of Udaipur.

Touny, E.M., El-Shobokshy, A.A. and El-Demerdash, O.M. 1976. The productive performance of lactating buffaloes fed different levels of concentrate. Agric. Rs. Rev., UAR: 54:9-14 (fide Dairy Sci. Abst., 40:5465).

Trung, L.T. and Gonzales, R.E. 1978. Organoleptic acceptance of fresh caraboo milk. Philippine J. Nutr., 31:36-40 (fide Dairy Sci. Abst. L, 40:2226).

Vishweshwaraiah, L. 1979. Studies on paneer. M.Sc. Thesis, Univ. Agric., Sci., Bangalore.

Waghmare, P.S. 1977. Srikhandagola. A new milk basd sweet meat. Indian Dairyman, 29:759-760.

Yegna Narayan Aiyer, A.K. 1953. Indian Dairyman, 5:63-77.

□□□

5

Buffalo Meat (Buffen) and Meat Products

Introduction

The edible part of carcass is known as meat. It is mainly flesh along with associated adipose tissue and some bones. Edible offal a glands like liver, kidneys, tongue, brain and knuckles *etc.*of buffaloes are also included in the market meat. Buffalo meat is consumed by a considerable population of Indian subcontinent, Egypt, Arabian countries, Italy, Bufarlia, Burma, Thailand, China, Laos, Kambodia, Vietnam, Philippines, Indonesia, Malayasia and many other countries. Buffaloes are primarily kept for milk and work in different countries and meat production is largely form the culled animals. Buffalo fattening is developing at a faster rate due to continuous increasing demand of edible meat. Protectie measures are being adopted for reducing the high calf mortality in buffaloes so that the spared male calves of dairy buffaloes may be finished as a good meat animalsof 300-400 kg body weight at about 12-18 months of age. Buffalo veal has a great demend a low fat, light coloured meat is more acceptable (Ferrara *et al.,* 1963; Franciscis *et al.,* 1970). The larger proportion of buffaloes are found in the agriculturally and economically developing countries probably due to their adaptability in the agroclimatic conditions of the tropical and sub-tropical zones. Although substantial information on various aspects of buffalo production have been published in recent years, indeed some miconcepts are carried by many people regarding the feeding and management of buffloes. Some recent litratures presented the scope of buffalo fattening on crop residues without much supplemental feeding. Probably such information is based on where say and theoretical assumptions. For obtaining optimum growth of about 500 g. daily for fininshing the male calves at 300 kg body weight, a palatable ration containing 8-10 percent digestible crude proteion and 60-65 per cent total digestible nutriens is required (Pathak *et al.*, 1982; Baruah *et al.*, 1983; pathak, 1966). Such high levels of digestible crude protein and energy could not be obtained by feeding inferior quality feeds and fodders. Buffaloes of high growth potential are not uncommon and average growth rate of 0.70 to 1.2 kg has been obtained on the feeding of high energy balanced diets (Avalisvili, 1956; Dzafarov, 1958; Kassir *et al.*, 1969; Taha *et al.*, 1980). Most of the recognized breeds of riverine and swampt bufflaoes are heavy animals of high growth poteintal buffalo fattening programme usually does not required breeding. Large scale fattening programme protecting male calves of dairy buffaloes may be started in many countries provided adequate supply of reasonably good quality feeds and fodders is assured.

Growth Performance of Buffalo on Natural and Improved Pastures

The pastures found in buffalo tract are mostly unmanaged natural grass covers and provide inferior quality natural herbage for grazing during the longer part of the year. Schima and Cenchrus are the dominant grasses tropical region and they also grow in the hostile climatic conditions of semi-arid and some parts of arid zones. Great variations occur in the herbage density duing the different seasons being maximum in the humid hot season. The nutritional quality of pastures is also much better in humid hot season than in the dry hot and cold seasons. Large variation has been reported in the growth response of buffaloes grazed on natural and improved pastures of India (Upadhayay *et al.*, 1980; Siddiqui *et al.*, 1982) and Australia (Ford, 1978; Robetson *et al.*, 1982). Average growth rate of buffalo calves on natural pastures of mixed grasses in semi-arid climate has been found to be 0.22 kg against the dry matter intake at the rate of 2 per cent of body weight (Siddiqui *et al.*, 1982). Signinficatly higher growth rates viz. 0.333 kg daily on Schima dorminatn pasture and 0.439 kg on Cenchrus dominant pastures have been observed during the lush growth of many seasons in central part of india (Upadhayay *et al.*, 1980).

On the natural grass cover of Northern Australia very poor growth rate has been observed during the long duration pastureing exceeding

3 years. Average of daily gain in body weight of swamp buffaloes after weaning was 0.16 to 0.17 kg on native pature (Ford, 1978)_ which increased to 0.24 to 0.32 kg daily when native pasture was improved by the sowing of Pangola, Calopo and Stylos (Robertson *et al.*, 1982). The growth rate is significantly affected by the qualitative and quantative availability of forages and it ranged ffrom 0.15 kg in dry season (July-December) to 0.58 kg int eh wet season (October-May) in the northern territory of Austraila. Similarly, ad libitum feeding of chaffed elephant grass could support about 0.25 kg daily gain in body weight which increased to about 0.54 kg daily on the feeding of rice bran to replace almost half of the dry matter supplied by the elephant grass. The grass contained 7.5 to 12.1 per cent crude protein on dry matter basis during the feeding (Moran, 1983). About 300-500 g daily gain in body weight of riverine buffalo calves may be obtained on ad libitum feeding of highly palatable good quality mixed fodder of cereal and leguminous cops (Agarwal, 1974; Naidu and Raghavan, 1985). The concept of buffalo rearing for meat producotn on unmanaged natural pastures may be considered ill -conceived and from the results of recent studies, it is apparent that adequate supply of nutritious feeds and fodders is an important component of buffalo fattening industry.

Buffaloes Available for Meat Production

Bufalo meat production in a developing industry which has gained momentum during the last two decades. Organized rearing of buffaloes exclusively for meat produciotn is limited to some Euro-Asian countries. Egypt, Pakistan, China, some south-east Asian countries. Australia and West Indies. Recently, it is being introducted in India. Normally, following four types of bufflaoes are available for meat production.

i) Young pre-ruminant calves of both sexes born in the urban andsub-urban dairies of the Indina sub-continent largely die in the very young age of 2-4 weeks due to parital or complete starvation and negligence. These the potential meat animals.

ii) Growing male calves culled at the end of lactation period of 9-15 months in the rural areas. These are mostly poor animals of 70-100 kg body weight which can be grown to 300-400 body weight for slaughter on scientific feeding and management.

iii) Sterile females may be young heifers of 3-4 years or older animals with irreparable reproductive problems.

iv) Retired working buffaloes are normally spared after 15 years of age.

The culled working animals of last two categories (iii and iv) have mostly poor health and their meat quality can be improved by feeding high energy rations for a short duration of 3-4 months.

Pattern of Gain in Body Weight

Conspicuous effect of feeding and management occurs onteh gain in body weight of buffaloes. Good quality buffalo veal comparable with that of cattle veal can be produced on feeding high quality ration of milk, milk replacer and concentrate mixture alongwith good quality legume hay (Kalugin, 1933). Growing animal have great inherent potential andhalf kg or more than 1 kg daily gain in body weight is obtained during post weaning growth and and 300 kg body weight at slaughter may be obtained at 9 months to 2 years of age depending on the nutritional quality of the diets and management of the animals (Arora and Gupta 1962; Ragab *et al.*, 1966; Charles and Johnson, 1972; Taha *et al.*, 1980; Borghese *et al.*, 1981; Baruah *et al.*, 1983). Scope of significant improvement in the carcass of culled buffaloes through the feeding of high energy diets for a period of 3-4 months has been demonstrated (Avalisvili, 1956; Polikhronov *et al.*, 1979). The growth pettern of bufflaoes for meat production has been described in brief for the diffenent types of animals.

a) Daily weight gain of buffalo veal (Buffeal) calves

The growth rate of young calves is affected by body weight at birth, inherent growth potential, feeds and levels of feeding and management practices. Normally buffalo veal calves are fed at high level of whole milk containing high concentration o favailable energy and balanced protein for a period of 4 to 18 weeks. The buffeat (veal) calves are slaughterd at a body weigh to f60 to 150 kg in 4 to 18 weeks of life (Badreldin, 1955; Ferrara *et al.*, 1963; Zakhariev, 1973; Salem *et al.*, 1983). Frequently of feeding milk or milk replacer diets alongwith other feeds had significant effect on the gain in body weight which has been reported higher on three times daily feeding at bout 8 hours interval (Verma and Tomer, 1984). A higher rate of gain is usually observed onteh feeding of whole milk of buffalo than the cow's milk (ABou-Hussain and Rafat, 1962; Ferrara *et al.*, 1967).

b) Daily body weight gain in growing buffaloes

Large variation occurs in the growth pattern of weaned buffalo calves and rate of gain in body weight is mainly effected by the plane of nutrition, which varies with the feeding value of rations. The gain in body weight ranges from negative to more that 1 kg (johri *et al.*, 1982; Robertson *et al.*, 1982). Average daily gain in body weight ranges from 0.16 to 0.26 kg on poor natural pastures of semi-arid India. Australia and Malasia (Ford, 1978; Robertson *et al.*, 11982, Siddiqui *et al.*, 1982; Moran, 1983). Considerably higher growth rate of 0.33 to 0.44 kg daily may be obtained on relatively better pastures of Sri Lanka and central India during the monsoon season (Matsukawa *et al.*, 1976; Upadhayay *et al.*, 1980). It has been found difficult to maintain the growing buffalo calves on the feeding of inferior quality roughage like wheat bhoosa as a sole ration. Supplementation of 2 per cent or higher level of urea alone or mixed with low levels (7 to 14 per cent) of sugarcane molasses has been found to be fatal (Johri, *et al.*, 1982). On the feeding of low quality ration of urea molasses liquid di *et al.*, ongwith intact protein supplement, gain in body weight may be 0.2 to 0.3 kg daily (Pathak *et al.*, 1976; Pathak and Ranjhan, 1979). Relatively higher gain in body weight is obtained on the freechoice feeding of nutritious green fodders and hay of oats, berseem, Lucerne and maize in suitable combinations (AGarwal, 1974; Naidu and Raghavan, 1985). About 0. 4kg to more than 1 kg daily gain in body weight is obtained ont eh feeding of conventional rations of concentrate mixture and fodder and rate of gain is significantly influenced by the feeding value of ration (Das Gupta, 1943; Tantwy, 1948; Cumburidge and Dalakisvili, 1959; Sharma and Talapatra, 1963; Ivanov and Zahariev, 1966; Ragab *et al.*, 1966; Kassir *et al.*, 1969; Juma *et al.*, 1972; Romita *et al.*, 1978; Rosa and Creta, 1978; Taha *et al.*, 1980; Borghese *et al.*, 1981: Baruah *et al.*, 1982; Pathak *et al.*, 1982).

c) Daily weight gain in culled buffaloes

The feeding of culled buffaloes for meat production depends on the body condition of animals, availability of good quality feeds at a reasonable price and return on capital input from the sale of meat and byproducts. System of feeding high energy rations to culled buffaloes in poor health is followed in some countries for the improvement of carcass quality but limited recoreded information is available in the literature. In a fattening feeding for 120 days, 840 g daily gain occurred in the body weight of culled buffaloes of 7-11 years of age. The rate of gain varied from 580-870 g in male and 790-1080 g in female buffaloes (Avalisvili, 1956). In a second feeding trial, mean gain in body weight was 711 g and feeding increased the proportion of fatty tissue in the carcass (Palikhronov *et al.*, 1979).

Feed/Nutrietn Conversion Efficiency

Considerable information has accumulated in recent years onteh feed and nutrients utilization efficiency of buffalo for gain in body weight. Most of the studies were aimed at growth production for replacement daily or draught animals. Some information are also available on feeding for the production of different kinds of buffalo meat like buff-veal,buffen (or cara beef) and other meats.

Average feed intake from a ration of buffalo milk and feeds has been found to be equivalent to 4.29 Scandinavian feed units for 1 kg gain in live weight (Salerno, 1948). Whole milk reuiremetn for 1 kg gain in body weight was 6 kg and for 1 kg dressed buffl-veal was 9 kg (Badreldin, 1955). Cow milk can replace buffalo milk but intake of former milk is about 65.5 per cent more than the latter mil for each unit gain in body weight (Ferrara *et al.*, 1967). The requirement of whole milk and concentrate mixture per kg gain in body weight of young calves fattened upto 36 weeks of age hjad been 2.51 kg and 1.03 kg respectively, besides the ad libitum feeding of good quality fodders (Borghese *et al.*, 1981).

Dry matter intake per kg gain in the body weight of buffaloes during the post weaning period varied from 5 to 21 kg depending upon the quality of feed and duration of feeding (Agrawal 1974; Tilakaratne *et al.*, 1976; Pathak and Ranjhan, 1979; Pathak *et al.*, 1982; Baruah *et al.*, 1983). The intake of dry matter per unit gain in body weight decreases with the corresponding increase in the energy content of rations.

Implantation of oestradiol-progesterone implant (Synovex-S) significantly improved the feed intake, daily gain in body weight and mean feed intake per kg gain in body weight was 8.8 kg against 9.63 kg in non-implanted male buffalo calves (Ali *et al.*, 1983).

Egyption fattening buffloes of about 230, 360 and 450 kg mean body weigh tat 12, 18 and 24 months of age needed 8.4, 9.0 and 11.7 kg starch equivalent per kg gain in body weight, respectively (Ragab, *et al.*, 1966).

The requirement in terms of Scandinavian feed unit consumption per kg gain in body weight ranges from 6 to 9 kg for fattening buffaloes gaining at the rate of 0.7 to 0.9 kg daily (Porot and Landi, 1965; Ivanov and Zahaiev, 1966).The feed conversion efficiency is significantly les sand pasture feeding (9.1 FU per kg gain) due to lower energy content (Kasimov, 1971; Gadzhiev *et al.*, 1973). Fattening Bulgarian Murrah and their F1 crosses required 7.24, 7.77 and 7.25 oat feed units (OFU) per kg gain in body weight for 1024, 951 and 1035 g average daily gain in body weight, respectively (Ognjanovie *et al.*, 1970). Mean body weigh tranged from 374 to 401 kg at 11-116 months of age.

Requirement of tatal digestible nutrients (TDN) per kg gain in body weight ranges from 4.91 to 5.2 kg for buffaloes fattened on high plane of nutrition from birth to approximately 400 kg body weight (EL-Naggar *et al.*, 1972; Ahmed and El-SHazly, 1975). In case of residual male buffalo calves, TDN requirement varied between 4.00 to 5.55 kg per kg gain in body weigh tan d5.77 -7.15 kg per kg gain in carcass weight for finishing at 300 kg mean body weight and about 450-550 g average daily gain in body weight (Baurah *et al.*, 1982; Pathak *et al.*, 1982; Pathak , 1996).

For the improvement of carcass traints of spent buffaloes average requirement is about 12.2 feed units per kg gain in body weight on high plane of feeding to support about 711 g daily gain in the body weight (Polikhronov *et al.*, 1979).

Slaughter of Buffaloes

Slaugheter of buffaloes for meat production is completed in the following sequence:

1. Pre-slaughter preparation: Buffaloes for slaughter are put in a lairage near the abattoir to rest for 4 hours. The animal are starved for 24 hours but offered free choice fresh drinking water.
2. Pre-mortem inspection: Pre-mortem inspection includes general inspection, recording of respiration, pulse, rectal temperature fand natural orifices.

a) Respiration, temperature and pulse should be in the normal range.

b) Mucous membrane of natural orifices should be pink and bright and there should not e any abnormal secretion.

c) Body should be clean, smooth and free from cuts and bruises.

d) Bones should be intact and normal.

e) Animal should not be emaciated.

f) Palpable lymph glands like suprascapular lymph node should not be enlarged.

3. **Washing of the animals:** The bufflaoes are washed clean by running water or beneath the fountain. The body is scrubed clean with a bush of handful of long grass hay.

4. **Restrain of the animal:** The buffalo is secured properly with a rope at the place of slaughter.

5. **Studding of buffales:** The animals are stunned to inactivate brain for human sacrifice. Precussive stunning is normally performed with a captive bolt pistol. The place of application of the captive pistol slightly varies with the age of the buffaloes.

   a) In adult buffaloes the crossing point of two oblique lines running from inner (medial) canthus of eye to the base o fthe opposite horn. The mouth of the captive pistol is placed secured at right angle of the forehead and fired quickly.

   b) In case of buffeal (buffalo calves of veal age) the point of captive pistol firing is about 10 mm below the crossing point used for the adult buffaloes.

   c) In retired buffaloes, the point of firing is about 1.5 cm lateral from the middle of the nose breeze.

   d) Electrical stunning: The animal is stunned by the application of electric current with a stunning form with electric current at 220-440 volts. The animal falls senseless in few seconds.

Methods of slaughter

Human method of slaugher has been recommended for global acceptance but in many countries still ritual methods of buffalo slaughter are followed. The main ritual methods of slaughter followed in the Bhartiya sub-continent are (i) halal and (ii) jhatka method. In both methods stunning ins not practiced.

a) Halal method of buffalo slaughter: The cleaned buffalo issecured properly by tying the four legs with a rope. The heat and hind parts are secured tightly. The head is kept in a particular direction and wind pipe and large vessels are cut from the ventral side with a sharp knife the level of larynx but the animal is not decapitated and the spinal cord remains intact. It is considred that bleeding is more effective and keeping quality is longer.

b) Jhatka method of buffalo slaughter: The animal are slaughtered in standing positon. The cleaned animal is secured by several people. The head is kept stretched and slightly downwards. A sharp heavy sword, dao or Khukari is used to decapitate the animal with one stroke on the neck. In this system, nervous system is cut in few seconds and pain is not felt. However, imcomplete bleeding reduces keeping quality.

Modern method or scientific slaughter

The stages of slaughter include fasting, cleaning, securing, stunning and decapitation.

Bleeding: Bleeding is completed by hanging the carcass with head downwards.

Flying: Flying is done when carcass is still hot. Blowing of air in the subcutaneous layer makes flying much easy. The intact hide is removed, washed and dried or stored in cold storage for sengin to tanneries.

Evisceration: The carcass is cut along the mid loine on the ventral aspect. The rectum is pulled after detaching by a careful circular incision around the anus, squeezed empty and then tied by a knot. This is done to prevent oiling and contamination of carcass with enteric contents. The alimentary canal, reproductive organs and urinary blader are removed and kept separate along the carcass for inspectin. The carcass presented for postmortem inspection contains intact respiratory system, large lymph nodes, heart, loiver and kidneys.

Post mortem inspection: It is done by a meat inspector (a veterinarian) trained for carcass inspection for healthy edible meat supply.

Carcass Characteristics

The carcass characteristics of edible meat of large animals are usually presented as carcass yield, dressing percentage, carcass length, carcass compositon and yield of edible andnon-edible offals etc.

a) Carcass yield and dressing percentage

The weight of carcass varies largely due to body size and physical status of animal and slaughter. Average weight of carcass including edible offals like liver, kidneys, heart, mesenteric fat and tail may be about 40.4 kg at about 30-40 days of age. Average yield of edible parts, head and feet was 65.75, 7.32 and 5.03 per cent respectively (Badreldin, 1955). Average dressing percentage may be 55-72 per cent for properly fed buffalo veal calves o 7 to 18 weeks of age (Ferrara *et al.*, 1963; Ragab *et al.*, 1966; Minieri *et al.*, 1968; Rasheed, 1977). Average dressing percentage of male may be slightly higher than the female buffalo veal calves (Salerno, 1962).

Carcass yield is low for culled animals and veried from 38 to 59 per cent depending onteh body condition of the animals (Maymone, 1945 Saleno, 1948; Domingues, 1956; Kurbano, 1961; Ferrara, 1964; Rao, 1978). Feeding of culled buffaloes for 3-4 months on good rations improves carcass yield and mean dressing percentage has been found to be 47.8 to 50.2 per cent after 90-120 days finishing period (Avalisvili, 1956; Polikhronov *et al.*, 1970).

Dressing percentage may be affected by the age at slaughter, sex, plane of nutrition and quality of feeds etc. The effect of various factors except the plane of nutrition has been found to be quite variable in different studies. Increase in dressing percentage has been recorded with corresponding increase in post-weaning body weight (Table 5.1) of male and female bufflaeos (Maymone, 1942, 1945; Saleno, 1948; Ragab *et al.*, 1966; Afifi *et al.*, 1974; Zakhariev, 1973; Zeiden *et al.*, 1976).

Table 5.1 Effect of age on the carcass yield (Zeiden *et al.*, 1976).

Carcass yield	Age in montsh		
	15	18	24
Body weight (kg)	407.4	441.3	486.5
Carcass weight (kg)	195.8	220.8	249.8
Dressing (%)	48.1	50.3	51.4
Chi8lling loss (%)	3.0	1.5	1.6

Large variation has been presorted to dressing percentage due to sex (Table 5.2) for buffaloes reared under different managemental conditions.

Table 5.2. Effect of sex and age on dressing percentage.

Sex	Age (months)	Body weight (kg)	Dressing (%)	Reference
Male	6.12		45	Maymone, 1945
	12.18		47	
	Adult		52	
Female	6.12		46	
	12-18		46	
	Adult		48	
Bulls	1-11/2	74	60	Ragab *et al.*, 1966a,b
	6	158	57.2	
	12	230	53.7	
	18	359	57.6	
	24	449	52.7	
Steers	12	236	53.3	
	18	360	54.5	
	24	450	54.3	
Entire	30	617	55.9	Aiearelli *et al.*, 1975
	42	688	60.0	
Bulls	A	388	50.8	Valin *et al.*, 1984
Steers I	A-0.5	387	51.4	
Steers II	A-5.5	477	53.3	
Steers III	A-7.0	541	53.1	

Large differnece in dressing percentage of carcass may occur in the buffaloes of different breeds with significant difference in birth weight and adult body weight, but little variation is found in the animals of similar growth potential. Mean dressing percentage in local sinhalee buffalo and Murrah buffalo was 49.7 and 53.4 for animal reared on a dry zone pasture of Srilanka (Matrukawa *et al.*, 1976) but in Bulgarian, Murrah and their crosses was 53.7 and 54.1 for the animals fattned intensively on same rations for a period of 130 days (Ognjanovie *et al.*, 1970).

Plane of nutrition and density of digestible energy in the rations significantly affect the carcass yield and dressing percentage increase in carcass yield and dressing percentage has been observed to level of feeding and compotion of diets (Agarwal, 1974; Pathak and Ranjhan, 1979). Feeding of poor animals significantly improve carcass yield and dressing percentage (Table 5.3) which is significatly affected by the density of energy in the diets (Baruah *et al.*, 1982).

Table 5.3. Effect of protein and energy levels in the diets on dressing percentage.

Nutrients	Body weight (kg)	Carcass weight (kg)	Dressing (%)
At start	75	35.1	46.8
Low protein x low energy	294	166.0	56.5
Low protein x medium energy	297	175.2	59.0
Low protein x high energy	309	178.0	57.6
High protein x low energy 293	293	161.6	55.2
High protein x medium energy	306	173.6	56.7
High protein x high energy	298	186.2	62.5

b) Dissectible tissue ratio of carcass

The acceptability of edible carcass for human consumption is determined by the ratio of lean, dissectible fat and bone in the carcass. Large variation occurs in the liking of human being from different countries. People of high income group prefer to eat lean carcass while those of low income group engaged in heavy physical work like fatty carcass. Eye muscle area or the area of cross section of Longissimus dorsi muscle at 10th rib is considered a satisfactory indicator of muscle caontent in the carcass. The ratio of dissectible tissue in the carcass is mainly affected by age, sex, plane of nutrition and energy content of diets (Ognjanovie *et al.*, 1970; Zakharleve, 1973; Agarwal, 1974; Charles and Johnson, 1975; Ziearrelli *et al.*, 1975; Pathak *et al.*, 1982; Valin *et al.*, 1984). Since different carcass ssamples have been used in various studies (Table 5.4), the values may not be closely comparable indeed they are informative and may be used for determination of carcass quality.

Table 5.4. Percentage of dissectible tissue in the carcass of different buffaloes.

Sl.	Type of animal	Dissectible tissue (%)			Reference
		Muscle	Fat	Bone	
1.	**Bulgarian**	71.9	9.9	18.2	Ognjanovie *et al.*, 1970
	Murrah	70.1	9.9	20.0	
	Murrah x Bulgarian (F1)	69.4	11.4	19.2	
2.	**High concentrate rations**				
	a) High level feeding	55.0	26.2	17.6	Agarwal, 1974
	b) Medium level feeding	53.2	26.9	18.5	
	High roughage ration				
	a) High level feeding	57.5	19.2	20.8	Agarwal, 1974
	b) Medium level feeding	56.0	19.1	23.1	
3.	**Age 30 months**				
	a) Entire	70.3	9.1	14.4	Zicarelli *et al.*, 1975
	b) Castrated	68.5	10.1	15.6	
	Age – 40 months				
	a) Entire	59.6	10.9	13.6	
	b) Castrated	68.5	10.1	15.6	
4.	**Low protein x low energy**	62.9	15.8	21.3	Pathak *et al.*, 1982
	Low protein x high energy	62.3	17.0	19.0	
	High protein x low energy	61.9	16.9	21.0	
	High protein x high energy	62.4	16.6	21.0	
5.	**Bulls-Age A + 0.5 months**	54	24	22	Valin *et al.*, 1984
	Steers- Age A + 0.5 months	52	29	19	
	Steers- Age A + 5.5 months	52	29	17	
	Steers- Age A + 7.0 months	53	29	18	

6. *Buff veal and young calves			
At birth	66.1	0.7	Zakhariev, 1973
3 months	72.9	0.5	
6 months	76.0	3.5	
12 months	79.0	8.2	
18 months	81.5	9.0	

* Muscle including bones also in trimmed lean.

The carcasses of spent buffaloes are graded into 3 groups i.e. good, fair and poor on the basis of the profile of hind quarters. The profile of loin and shoulders is also considered (Kondaiah *et al.,* 1 981). Average meat percentage is higher in male than in the female buffaloes (Table 5.5). The ratio of bone increases with the decrease in conformation score of the carcasses of male buffaloes of same grade (Kondaiah *et al.,* 1983).

Table 5.5. Ratio of dissectible tissue in different grades of buffalo carcass.

Carcass grade	Sex	Percentage of dissectible tissue			
		Carcass weight (kg)	Muscle	Bone	Fat+Fascia
Good	Male	155.2	7.17	22.5	4.8
	Female	188.4	65.3	19.1	15.1
	Pooled	171.3	69.0	20.8	10.0
Fair	Male	157.7	68.1	26.5	5.4
	Female	178.7	67.5	22.7	9.8
	Pooled	168.1	67.8	24.6	7.6
Poor	Male	143.6	66.0	28.9	5.1
	Female	139.2	63.7	29.5	6.8
	Pooled	140.9	64.8	29.2	6.0

c) Meat: Bone ratio

Muscle and fat including fascia are considered together in the edible part of carcass although marrow of long bones is also used for the preparation of soup and other dishes. Wider meal: bone ratio indicates better finish and meatiness of the carcass. In addition to nutritional statues, the age, sex and conformation are the factors affection the meat:bone ratio of the carcass (Table 5.6). Meat content is higher in veal and young animals (Ferrara *et al.,* 1963; Romita *et al.,* 1978). Wider meat: bone ratio is normally observed int ehcarcasses of female and castrated buffaloes (Minieri *et al.,* 1972; Kondaiah *et al.,* 1983) and buffaloes fed high level of energy (Agarwal, 1974; Charles and Johnson, 1975; Pathak *et al.,* 1982).

Table 5.6. Effect of various factors on meal: bone ratio of carcass

Sl.	Factors		Meat:bone ratio	Reference
1.	Age	20 months	3.02	Romita *et al.,* 1978
		28 months	3.54	
		36 months	3.54	
2.	Sex	Bulls	3.97	Minieri *et al.,* 1972
		Steers	4.01	Kondaiah *et al.,* 1983
3.	Conformation			
	Good	Male	3.46	Kondaiah *et al.,* 1983
		Female	4.18	
	Fair	Male	2.78	
		Female	3.44	
	Poor	Male	2.47	
		Female	2.39	
4.	Feeding regime	All hay	4.08	CDharles and Johnson, 1975
		All pettels	4.48	
5.	Level of feed energy	Low	3.69	Pathak *et al.,* 1982
		High	4.04	

d) Eye muscle or Loin eye area

The area of longissimus dorst muscle commonly known as eye muscle or loin eye is a good indicator of meatiness of carcass. It is the area of a crosssection fo eye muscle between 12th and 13th rib. The eye muscle area is affected by age, sex, breed and carcass conformation (Table 5.7) but is aged animals it may not be very useful (Kondaiah *et al.,* 1983).

Table 5.7. Effect of various factors on the eye muscle area

Sl	Factors	Eye muscle area (cm²)	Reference
1. **Age and sex (bulls)**	50 days	24	Ragab *et al.*, 1966
	6 montsh	37	
	12 montsh	45	
	18 montsh	66	
	24 montsh	85	
2. **Sex**			
Castrated	12 montsh	40	
	18 montsh	63	
	24 montsh	75	
3. **Breed**	Bulgarian	64.3	Gnjanovie *et al.*, 1970
	Murrah	60.6	
	Murrahx Bulg. (F1)	63.4	
4. **Plane of nutrition**	Poor weaned calf	11.3	Baruah, 1982
	Low protein - low energy	41.9	
	Low protein - medium energy	49.4	
	Low protein - high energy	50.6	
5. **Carcass grade**	Good	23.5	Kondiah *et al.*, 1983
	Fair	21.9	
	Poor	20.4	

e) Carcass cutability characters

For retain sale carcass is normally dissected into various cuts to satisfy the requirement of consumers. Retail cuts of buffalo carcass vary largely between countries and standard cuts are mostly undefined local terms which vary significantly from place to place. Some information available ont eh carcass cutability (Table. 5.8) according to cuts of beef described by Ziegler (1964) provide valuable information about the properly funished buffen (Agarwal, 1974; Baruah, 1982).

Table 5.8. Cutability characters of carcass (%)

Carcass traits	High concentration ration	High fodder ration
Neck	4.13	4.98
Chuck	17.43	18.33
Fore shank	5.25	5.11
Brisket	6.30	6.42
Plate	6.37	6.63
Rib	10.17	10.61
Loin	14.97	15.99
Rump	5.47	7.21
Round	22.35	20.33
Hind shank	5.03	2.49

Edible Offals

Various organs, head and tongue are also consumed by the human beings and they are included in edible meat in many countrei. Yield of edible offals mainly depends on breed, body weight anc condition of the animal (Kassir *et al.*, 1969, Ognjanovie *et al.*, 1970; AGarwal, 1974; Pathak *et al.*, 1982; Kondaiah *et al.*, 1983; Lakshmanan *et al.*, 1984). Edible offals of buffalo carcass may be classified as follows:

a) **Offal meat:** Heaat meat, oesophagus meat, diaphragm meat, knuckles meat and tail meat.

b) **Edible organs:** Liver, kidneys, brain, heart, udder and teats, tongue, testis, lungs and wind pipe, spleen and gastro-intertinal tract.

c) **Offal fat:** Caul fat, mesenteric fat.

d) **Blood:** Whoel blood, cloth and serum.

In addition to these skin pieces removed from the hip region are also used for the preparation of special dishes in Philippines and other countries of the region. Yield of various edible organs in different types of buffaloes shows great variation (Table 5.9). Buffaloes with logn horns had higher proportion of heat in body weigh than the short horn varieties. Similarly, ratio of many organs is higher in poor than in healthy animal.

Table 5.9. Proportion of edible offals in the live weight of buffaloes.

Organs	Iraqi buf-falo	Bulga-rian buffalo	Murrah buffalo	Murrah x bulga-rian (F1)	Indian desi	Swamp buffalo	Buf-falo veal
Body weight (kg)	335	376	374	401	298.312	300	61
% of body weight Head	4.06	3.87	3.66	3.91	5.91-6.37	58	7.32
Feet/knuckles	2.36	1.95	1.99	1.83	1.91-1.07	2.9	5.03
Liver	1.41	1.12	1.15	1.12	0.73-0.89	1.4	-
Kidney	0.27	0.20	0.26	0.17	0.20-0.21	-	-
Heart	0.41	0.36	0.43	0.37	0.31-0.37	0.6	-
Tongue	-	0.23	0.27	0.19	-	-	-
Spleen	-	-	-	-	0.20-0.25	'0.2	-
Lungs		0.52	0.56	0.49	-	-	1.26
Blood	-	-	-	-	3.83-4.01	-	-

Some characterisitics of Muscle Tissue

The structural units of muscles are muscle fibres which are long, slender cells containing several nuclei. The diameter rof muscle fibre is affected by age, sex, breen, plane of nutrition and exercise. Variation in physical and chemical characteristics of muscle tissue (Tables 5.10 and 5.11) has been observed for different breeds (Ognjanovie *et al.*, 1970), body condition (rao, 1978), age (Yadav, 1982), body weight and sex at finishing (Valin *et al.*, 1984) and fibres of the muscles (Soloman *et al.*, 1985).

Table 5.10. Some chemical and physical characteristics of muscle tissue

Factors	Moist-ure (%)	Protein (%)	Lipids (%)	Myoglo bin(%)	Oxy-proline (%)	Muscle fibre	Buffalo veal
						Popula-tion (%)	Diameter (μ)
Poor animals of							
60-69kg	78.46	18.82	1.52	-	-	-	33.37
100-130 kg	76.38	18.90	1.27	-	-	-	41.07
140-160 kg	78.27	18.59	1.24	-	-	-	28.89
Breeds							
Bulgarian	-	-	-1.36	1.53	0.78	-	58.73
Murrah (Bulg)	-	-	0.64	1.40	10.74	-	57.14
Murrah x Bulg.	-	-	1.04	1.37	0.70	-	56.67
Fibre type							
		i) At 14 montsh (372 kg)					
a) Red	-	-	-	-	-	20.7	28.98
b) Intermediate	-	-	-	-	-	79.7	38.29
		ii) At 7 years (675 kg)					
a) Red	-	-	-	-	-	26.3	51.15
b) Intermediate	-	-	-	-	-	73.7	58.34

Table. 5.11. Effect of age and finishing body weight on physico-chemical characterists of muscle tissues in some muscles

Body weight (kg)	Muscle	Mois-ture (%)	Protein (%)	Lipids (%)	Glyco-gen (%)	pH	Myogl-obin (%)	Muscle fibre Dia (μ)
Bull								
388	Longissi-mus dorsi	75.5	23.1	1.8		5.6	2.9	-
Steers								
387	-do	75.4	22.7	1.7	-	5.6	2.7	-
477	-do-	74.5	22.6	1.6	-	5.8	3.8	-
541	-do-	74.9	23.0	1.5	-	5.9	3.7	-
Bulls								
a) 1 yr, 160	-do-	78.2	16.61	-	1.19	5.91	-	44.65
b) 2 yr, 289	-do-	77.5	17.01	-	1.28	5.95	-	57.16
c) 3 yr, 367	-do-	76.5	17.26	-	0.96	5.83	-	65.32

d) 5 yr, 498	-do-	75.7	19.21	-	0.90	6.10	-	89.19
(A)	Biceps branchei	78.8	16.70	-	-	5.95	-	42.56
(B)	-do-	77.3	16.85	-	1.17	5.99	-	57.68
(C)	-do-	76.6	17.54	-	0.95	5.87	-	64.60
(D)	-do-	75.7	19.45	-	1.01	6.10	-	84.86
(A)	Semi-ten dinosus	78.5	16.61	-	1.05	5.83	-	44.95
(B)	-do-	77.3	17.23	-	1.17	5.96	-	58.67
(C)	-do-	76.7	17.30		1.00	5.82	-	68.89
(D)	-do-	75.8	19.29		1.00	6.01	-	91.77

Chemical composition of Meat

Buffalo meat contains relatively more proteion and less lipid thatn the beef at similar level of growth. Protein content is higher in lean meat and bones of the carcass than in the fatty tissue (AGarwal, 1974). The chemical compositoni of meat is affected by the age, sex, breed, degree of fattening, compositon of diets and use of growth hormones and biostiumulators (Kurbanov, 1961; Ferrara *et al.,* 1969; Franciscis *et al.,* 1970; Rao, 1978). Normally proportion of moisture decreases and that of fat increases with the increase in age and degree of fatness (Table 5.12) through the feeding of high energy diets.

Table 5.12. Chemical composition of buffalo meat (%).

Type of meat	Moisture	Protein	Fat	Ash	Energy Kcal/ kg
Buff veal	73.02	20.84	4.30	0.97	1230
Buff eal-on					
Buffalo milk	71.68	21.41	5.83	1.04	1400
Cow milk	73.15	20.37	5.35	1.01	1400
Light weight	70.70	21.00	7.24	0.97	1515
Fatty carcass	64.42	19.18	15.40	1.00	2556
Medium carcass	68.87	20.50	9.60	1.03	2080
Lean carcass	73.35	22.40	1.15	1.08	1386
Poor carcass	77.70	18.77	1.43	-	-
High energy feed					
Muscle tissue	68.20	24.34	6.06	1.56	1540
Bone tissue	36.73	22.74	11.85	28.68	2006
Fat tissue	13.55	3.65	82.56	0.31	778

Amino Acid Content of Meat

Amino acid content in meat of different buffalo breeds (Table (5.13) Shows reasonable difference in the protein (Ognjanovic *et al.*, 1970).

Table 5.13. Amino acid content in fresh Longissimus dorsi muscle (%).

Amino acids	Bulgarian	Murrah (Bulgaria)	Murrah x Bulgarian (F1)
Alanine	1.416	1.571	1.488
Arginine	1.218	1.435	1.422
Aspartic acid	2.555	2.518	2.625
Cystine	0.363	0.523	0.544
Glycine	1.066	1.963	0.544
Glutamic acid	3.965	4.311	4.154
Histidine	0.767	0.868	0.835
Isoleucine	1.227	1.159	1.233
Lysine	1.800	2.162	1.722
Methionie	0.646	0.660	0.659
Phenylaline	0.904	0.955	0.966
Proline	1.185	0.914	0.928
Serine	0.874	0.899	0.926
Threonine	1.172	1.186	1.231
Tyrosine	0.816	0.871	0.894
Valine	1.318	1.370	1.355

The amino acids in F1 Murrahx Bulgarian crossbred buffalo meat show variable genetic effect but in most cases it was in between the two parent breeds. Amino acids composition of skeletal muscle of water buffalo, ox and African buffalo (Table 5.14) indicates the protein richness of buffalo meat (Cutinelli-Ambesi *et al.*, 1975).

Table 5.14. Amino acid content of skeletal muscle (A=mg per g dried meat and B=g per 100 g of amino acids)

Amino acids	Buffalo		African buffalo		Ox	
	A	B	A	B	A	B
Alanine	52.6	6.3	62.4	6.4	35.6	7.5
Arginine	56.8	6.8	69.7	7.1	27.9	5.9
Aspartic acid	89.4	10.7	82.5	8.4	47.9	10.2
Glutamic acid	142.8	17.1	132.4	13.5	70.6	15.0
Glycine	34.2	4.1	44.3	4.5	21.0	4.5
Histodine	29.2	3.5	29.5	3.0	15.5	3.3
Isoleucine	46.8	5.6	52.5	5.4	27.5	5.8
Leucine	76.0	91.	102.3	10.4	42.0	8.9
Lysine	79.4	9.5	81.9	8.4	38.0	8.1
Methionine	23.4	2.8	35.8	3.7	14.9	3.2
Phenylalanine	34.2	4.1	46.3	4.7	24.8	5.3
Proline	27.6	3.3	41.4	4.2	16.1	3.4
Serine	35.1	4.2	45.2	4.6	21.0	4.5
Threonine	35.9	4.3	48.8	5.0	23.8	5.0
Tyrosine	29.2	3.5	48.9	5.0	21.7	4.6
Valine	42.6	5.1	55.1	5.6	23.4	5.0

The amino acids composition of the sarcoplasmic, myofibrillar and insoluble fractions of skeletal muscle proteins shows higher solubility of histidine, valine, leucine, tyrosine, phenylalanine and methionine (Table 5.15) in domestic buffalo (Colonna *et al.*, 1975).

Table 5.15. Amino acid composition of different fractions of skeletal muscle protein of domestic buffalo (% per 100 g protein)

Amino acids	Sarcoplasmic protein	Myofibrillar protein	Insoluble protein
Alanine	6.1	7.9	9.1
Arginine	4.9	6.7	7.6
Aspartic acid	9.0	10.4	9.8
Glutamic acid	11.9	18.4	17.5
Glycine	5.0	3.9	12.4
Histidine	7.8	2.5	1.8

Isoleucine	5.9	6.1	5.4
Leucine	12.1	10.8	8.0
Lysine	11.7	10.2	8.0
Methionine	3.9	3.8	2.8
Phenylalanine	5.8	4.8	4.1
Proline	3.0	2.7	7.5
Serine	4.2	4.8	3.1
Threonine	5.2	5.8	4.2
Tyrosine	4.3	3.5	3.7
Valine	7.4	5.2	5.7

Slaughter Byproducts

Average carcass yield ranges from 40 to 60 per cent of the body weight at slaughter and the remaining portion is byproducts. Slaughter byproducts include edible and non-edible offals and a large amount of gastrointestinal fill. Edible byproducts are blood, liver, heart, spleen, lungs including wind pipe, head, feet and emply gastro-intestinal tract after proper cleaning and processing. Edible byproducts yield varies from 10-12 per cent of live weight depending upon the condition of animal. Non-edible by byproducts are the hide, horns, hooves, hairs and gut fill. Average yield of various byproducts has beenfound to be higher (Table 5.16) for the animals of mostly poor to fair conformation slaughtered inmany countries of the tropical buffalo tract (Kondaiah *et al.,* 1983).

Table 5.16. Yield of byproducts in slaughtered buffaloes

Byproducts	Range (kg)	Mean (kg)	Per cent yield
Hide	34-70	47.0	13.62
Head	15-21	17.3	5.02
Pluck	4-9	6.3	1.83
Blood	7-13	9.5	2.76
Feet	5-7	6.1	1.76
Horns	0.92-3.2	1.9	0.55
Liver	2.7-5.8	4.3	1.26
Spleen	0.6-1.2	1.0	0.29
Kidneys	0.8-1.1	1.0	0.29
Brain	0.4-0.5	0.5	0.13

Caul fat	2.3-7.3	4.7	1.37
Rumen	5.4-10.4	7.5	2.18
Reticulum	1.1-2.1	1.6	0.47
Omasum	0.9-3.8	2.8	0.80
Intestine	8-21	15.5	4.49
Mesentery	4.6-8.0	6.0	1.74
Rumen content	20-67	42.4	12.28

Meal Products

Edible buffalo meats include primal carcass cuts and edible offals. Primal cuts are used for the preparation of standard dishes popoular in different countries, while edible offals are sually made into minced meat (keema). The primal cuts are sold at retain shops. Since availability of meat is inadequate for human consumption inmost of the buffalo raising coutries, little attempt has been made for the development of preserved meat products. Offal meats commonly referred as variety meats include meats separated from the head, feet, pluck, oesophagus, rumenand upper half of the diaphragm. These are chopped finely and then mixed to make keema. Prepartions of keema are quite popular in the Indian sub-continent which include keema curry, pakoda, kofta, tikki, kabab and seekh kabab etc. These preparations are made after mixing chili, condiments, garlic, onion and salt according to tast and then fried in boiling oil or fat except the curry is cooked in usual manner to contain sufficient soup and seekh kabab is cooked hanged on the direct slow heat of charcoal.

Some Local Meat Products of Different Countries

Although surplus meat is not available for preservation, indeed some people prepare special products for consumptions at specific occasions.

Products of Indian sub-continent

1. **Dired Salted meat:** Fresh mat is cut into strips of 1-2 cm thickness, powdered common salt is thoroughly rubbed with the meat strips. The salt is used at the rate of 3-5 per cent of the raw meat. Salted meat is prepared on clean cloth or polyethylene sheet for sun drying. Meat is dried to less than 10 per cent moisture content in 3-4 days when good sun light is available for 8-10 hours daily. Dried salted meat is used during the scarcity period

and at remote places where cats are not available. It is washed in fresh water before cooking in the usual manner.

2. **Dried masala meat:** Raw meat is cut into pieces of 1-2 cm2 and mixed with a paste of onion, garlic, condiments and 2-3 percent salt. The salted masala meat is sun dried for 3-4 days to contain less thatn 10 percent moisture. Dried masala meat is a ready to cook material available in some homes and preferably fried in boiling oil for eating as snacks.

Products of Turkey

Steak and sausages are popular in Turkey.

Products of Indonesia

1. **Sun dried meat:** strips of raw meat are rubbed with blood and then sun dried for use as biltong or jerked meat. The process is more popular in Bali island.
2. **Kerupuk kulti:** is prepared form the hides of hip region after scrapping and cleaning in boiling water.
3. **Djingur:** is prepared from the lips.

Products of Philipines

Chicharones or cracklings are prepared fromteh hide of hips removed alongwith tail. The another common product in kari-kari.

Products or Thailand

Three hide products namely khab-kwai, nung-pong and chin - pong are quite common in the northern Thailand. They are prepared by boiling, salting and drying of hide strips and cooked as curry or fried in boiling fat.

Modern meat products

Works are in progress for developing the processes for the preparation of modern meat products of buffalo meat. An acceptable recipe for buff sausage has been developed at the Indian Veterinary Research Institute, Izatnagar (Sharma *et al.*, 1982). Other Indian products popular in consumers are seekh kabab, kofta, tikka, nuggests *etc.*

References

Abou-Hussein, E.R.M. and Rafat, M.A. 1982. Comparative studies on the feeding of dairy buffalo calves on cow's and buffalo's milk. J. Anim, Prod. UAR, 2:27-33.

Afifi, Y.A. Shain, M.A., Omara, S.F. and Youssef, F.M. 1974. Meat production from buffalo. Agril. Res. Rev., 52(7):1-15.

Agarwal, V.P. 1974. Studies on growth rate and carcass quality of buffalo calves as influenced by different planes of nutrition. Ph.D. Thesis. Agra University, Agra.

Ahmed, I.A.a nd El-Shazly, K. 1975. Early weaning of buffaloes in Egypt. World Anim. Rev., 14:26-30.

Ali, A., Cheema, A.U., Mirza and Alvi, A.S. 1983.The effect of synovex-S the performance and carcass quality of male buffalo calves. Buffalo Bulletin, 4:55.

Arora, S.P.a nd Gupta, B.S. 1962. Some factors affecting the growth rate of Murrah buffalo calves. J. Vet., Anim. Husb. Res., MHOW, 6: 19-21.

Avalisvili, N. 1956. The fattening of buffaloes. Moloch. Myasn. Zhiv., 8:60-61 (fide Anim. Breed. Abstr., 25:58).

Badreldin, A.L. 1955. Dressing out percentage in suckling buffalo veals. Indian J. Vet. Sci., Anim. Husb., 25:58).

Badreldin, A.L. 1955. Dressing out percentage in suckling buffalo veals. Indian J. Vet. Sci. Anim. Husb., 25:58.

Baruah, K.K., Rajhnan, S.K. and Pathak, N.N. 1982. Effect of various levels of protein and energy feeding on growth, digestibility of organic nutrients and carcass characterisctics of Indian desi male buffalo calves.

Borghese, A., Romita, A., Singli, S. and Marchini, S. 1981. Comparative trial on bovine and buffalo calves. 1. Daily gain, food conversion efficiency and carcass data from animals at 36 weeks of age. Annali dell Inst. Sper. Zootecnia, 12(1): 63 (fide Anim. Breed. Abstr., 49: 44-48).

Charles, D.D. and Johnson, E.R. 1972. Carcass composition of the water buffalo (*Bubalus bubalis*). Austrialian J. Agric., Res., 23: 905-911.

Colonna, G., Iracė, G., Balestrieri, C., Minieri, L. and Salvatore, F. 1975. Amino acid composition of skeletal muscle of domestic buffalo (*Bas bubalis*). II, Fractions in three protein fraction and studies on their amino acid pattern, Comp. Biochem. Physiol., 51(B):197-200.

Cumburidze, S. and Dalakisvili, G. 1959. The effectiveness of fattening bufflaoes kept partly indoor. Moloch. Mayasn. Zhiv., 4:16-18 (fide Anim. Breed. Abstr., 28:81).

Cutinelli-Ammbesi, L., Bocchini, V., Balestrieri, C. and Slavatore, F. 1975. Amino acid composition of skeletal muscle of domestic buffalo (*Bos bubalis*). I. Comparative studies and nutritional values of proteions. Comp. Biochem. Physiol., 51(B):193-196.

Das Gupta, N.C. 1943. Indian J. Vet., Sci., Anim. Husb., 13:196.

Domingues, O. 1956. The buffaloes in Brazil. Anim. Agril. Bras., 3(9): 15-21.

Dzafarov, S. 1958. Buffalo Breeding- A valuable source of butter and meat production. Motoch. Myasn. Zhiv., 3:16-19 (fide Anim. Breed. Abstr., 36:1820).

El-Naggar, A.A.., El-Shazly, K. and Ahmed, I.A. 1972. Effect of early weaning on the performance of male buffalo and cattle calves. Anim. Prod., 14:171-176.

Ferrara, B. 1964. The present situation of buffalo breeding in Italy. Acta. Med. Ver. Napali, 10:325-355.

Ferrara, B., Minieri, L. and Franciscis, G. De., 1967. Feeding buffalo calves on buffalo and cow milk. Atti. Soc. Ital. Sci. vet., 21:441-445.

Ford, B.D. 1978. Live weight changes of swamp buffaloes and cattle in Northern Australia. M.Sc. Dissertation. Centre for Tropical Veterinary Medicine, University of Edinburg, Great Britain.

Franciscis, G. De., Interieri, F., Rinaldi, G. and Rendin, N. 1970. Chemical analysis of the meat and components of the fifty edible quarter of early weaned buffalo calves and young light weight buffaloes. Atti della Soc. Ital. Sci. Vet., 24:349-351 (fide Anim. Breed. Abstr. 41:43).

Gadzhiev, G.K. Yusupov., K.Y.a nd Kasimov, M.H. 1973. Fattening and slaughter characters of young buffaloes and simental cattle in Dagestan. Zhivotnovodstvo, 10:75-77 (fide Anim. Breed. Abstr., 42:925).

Ivanov, P.a nd Zahariev, Z. 1966. The fattening ability of buffaloes. Nauchini Trud. Vissh. Sels. Inst. Georgi. Dimitrov. Zootek. Fak., 16:113-122 (Fide Anim. Breed. Abstr., 35:3347).

Johri, C.B., Ranjhan, S.K. and Pathak, N.N. 1982. Effect of different levels of molasses substitution on 205 per cent urea impregnated wheat bhoosa on the voluntary intake, digestibility of nutrients and growth response of male buffalo calves (*bubalus bubalis*). Indian J. Anim. Sci., 42:192-198.

Jul, M. and Padda, G.S. 1984. Meat producton in India: The potential of buffalo beef. World Anim. Rev., 50:36-44.

Juma, K.H., Farhan, S.M.A. and Faraj, M. 1972. Feed lot performance of native cow and buffalo calves in Iraq. Indian J. Anim. Sci., 42: 406-411.

Kalugin, I.I., 1933. The buffalo. Probl., Zhivotn., 1:57-58 (fide Anim. Breed. Abstr., 1:89).

Kavimov, M. 1971. Fattening performance of buffaloes in Dagestan. Molach. Myas, Skotovod., Mosk., 16:14 (fide Anim. Breed. Abstr., 40:130).

Kondaiah, N., Lakshmanan, V., Rao, V.K. and Sharma, N. 1981. Studies on type and conformation of slaughter buffaloes and carcass in India. Indian J. Anim. Res, 15:107-111.

Kondaiah, N., Lakshmanan, V., Anjaneyulu, A.S.R. and Sharma, N. 1983. Evaluation of aged and spent buffaloes for meat. Indian J. Anim. Sci, 53:1208-1212.

Kurbanov, I. 1961. A study of buffalo meat quality. Miasnaia Industrija, SSSR, Mosk, 5:47049.

Lakshmanan, V., Kondaiah, N. and Anjaneyulu, A.S.R. 1984. Variety meats of buffalo. Buffalo Bulletin, 3:6-8, 17.

Matsukawa, T., Tilakratne, N. and Bhuvanendran, V. 1976. Growth and carcass characteristics of cattle and buffalo breed on a dry zone pature in Srilanka (Ceylon). Tropical Anim. Hlth. Prod., 8:155-162.

Maymonc, B. 1942. Buffalo in Italy, Z., Tierzucht. Zuchtbiol., 51:1-44.

Maymone, B. 1945. Rearing buffaloes in Italy. Amali 1st Scrp. Zootech., Roma, 3:5-65.

Minieri, L., Franciscis, G. De, Interieri, F. and Richetchi, F. 1969. Slaughter yield of buffalo calves fed on reconstituted milk. Acta. Med. Vet. Napalai, 14:59-70 (fide Anim. Breed. Abstr., 37:1268).

Minieri, L., Franciscis, G De., Barbieri, V. and Zicarelli, L. 1972. Slaughter tests of entire buffaloes. Acta med., Vet., Napali, 18:19-33(fide Anim. Breed. Abstr., 41:2500).

Moran, J.E. 1983. Rice bran as a supplement to elephant grass for cattle and buffalo in Indonesia. I. Feed intake, utilization and growth rate. 2. Carcass development, energy accretion and its effects on feed efficiency. J. Agril., Sci., UK, 100:709-722.

Naidu, M.M. and Raghavan, G.B. 1985. Effect of plane of nutrition on growth in male Murrah buffaloes. Indian Vet. J, 62:64-70.

Ognjanovie, A., Polikhronov, D. and josksimovie, JU. 1970. The possibility of improving the yield and quality of buffalo meat by crossing. Proc. Meat of Meat Research Workers, Sofia, Bulgaria, Sept., 1970.

Pathak, N.N. 1985. Growth response and carcass yield of desi male buffalo calves finished on and libitum feeding of urea molasses liquid diet with restricted oats forage and intact protein supplement. Proc., Nat. Symp. 'Use of Nuclear Technique Anim. Health Prod.', pp. 15, Indian Veterinary Research Institute, Izatnagar.

Pathak, N.N. and Ranjhan, S.K. 1979. Growth response of male buffalo calves on different plane of nutrition. Proc. Protein and NPN utilization in ruminants. Pp. 10-11. National Dairy Research Institute, Karnal.

Pathak, N.N.,Krishna Mohan, D.V.G. and Ranjhan, S.K. 1976. A note on the Voluntary intake and growth response of buffalo calves fed and lib urea molasses liquid diet and restricted cereal forage with different supplementary nitrogenous feeds. Indian J. Anim. Sci., 46:451-453.

Pathak, N.N., Baruah, K.K. and Ranjhan, S.K. 1982. Nutrients utilization and carcass characteristics of male buffalo calves on different planes of nutrition.

Polikhronov, D., Boikovski, S. and Pinkas, A., 1979. Fattening buffalo cows culled from reproduction. Zhivotnov 'dni Nauki', 16(8):15-20 (fide Anim. Breed., Abstr., 49:2488).

Proto, V. and Landi, F. 1965. Meat production tests with young buffalo bulls. Poduz. Anim. 4:237-242 (finde Anim. Breed. Abstr., 34:1048).

Ragab, M.T., Darvish, M.Y.H. and Malam, A.G.A. 1966a. Meat production from Egyptian bufflaoes. I. Developomental changes and dressing percentage in a group of buffalo males. J. Aim. Prod., UAR, 6:9-30.

Rao, B.R. 1978. Preliminary studies on certain quantitative and qualitative characteristics of buffalo meat. Indian Vet. J., 55:111-118.

Rasheed, A.A. 1977. A preliminary investigation on the relationship between some linear body measurements and body live and dressed carcass weights of male buffalo vealers raised in Egypt. Libyan j. Agril., 6:269-274 (fide Anim. Breed., Abstr., 47:3483).

Robertson, J.A., Ford, B.D. and Morris, C.A. 1982. Live weight changes in carcass measurement in buffalo (*Bubablus bubalis*) and brahmanx

Northern territory short horn (Bos indicus x Bos taurus) Stters Upto 4 years of age grazing on improved pastures. Australian J. Agril., Res., 33: 755-762.

Romita, a., Borghese, A., Gigli, S. and Giacomo, A.D. 1978. Growth rate and carcass composition of water buffalo calves and bovine calves slaughtered at 20, 28 and 36 weeks. Proc. Seminar on pattern of Growth and Development in Cattle, Netherlands, Hague, pp. 523-534 (fide Anim. Breed. Abstr., 47:5331).

Rosa, A. and Creta, V. 1978. The value of young buffaloes for meat production- an important reserave for increasing meat production. Revista Decreastera Anim., 28(10):9-13 (fode Anim. Breed. Abstr., 47:5910).

Salerno, A. 1948. Meat production from buffaloes reared in Italy. Annali Fac. Agril., Univ. Bari., 6:51-96.

Salem, M.A.I., Nigam, A.A. and abdel-Aziz, A.S. 1983. Changes in carcass characteristics of Egyptian buffaloes during the first six months of age Egyptian J. Anim. Prod., 23:77-78 (fide Anim. Breed. ABstr., 52:6337).

Sharma, K.M. and Talapatra, S.K 1963. Growth response in buffalo calves. Indian J. Dairy Sci. 16:236-244.

Sharma, N., Padda, G.S. and Kondaiah, N. 1982. Preparation of buffalo Sausages. Indian food Packer, 50-52.

Siddiqui, I.A., Maheshwari, M.L. and Barsaul, C.S. 1982. Nutrition of buffalo calves on pasture. Vet. Res. J., 5:71-72.

Solomon, M.B., West, R.L. and carpenter, J.W. 1985. Fibre types in the longissimus muscle from water buffalo and selected domestic beef breeds. Meat Sci. 13:129-135.

Taha, Z., Zeiden, M., Roushey, S.A. and Sedik, M.F. 1980. Developomental changes in male buffalo calves. Asscrit. Vet Med. J., 6:191-199 (fide Anim. Breed. Abstr., 49:1190).

Tantawey, A.O. 1948. Growth in Egyptian cattle. Thesis. Facultry of Agril. Farouk. I. Univ., Alexandria.

Tilakratne, N., Matsukawa, T., Buvanendran, V. and Thangarajah, P. 1976. Growth, feed conversion and carcass characteristics of cattle and buffloes fed grass and concentrates. Ceylon Vet. J., 24:9-12.

Upadyayay, V.S. and Rai, P. and Patil, B.D. 1980. Comparison of two tropical grass species for growth and milk production in dairy cattle under grazing conditions. Indian J. Range Mgmt., 1:129-135.

Valin, C., Pinkas, A., Dragnev, H., Boikovski, S. and Polikhronov, D. 1984. Comparative study of buffalo meat and beef. Meat Sci., 10: 80-84.

Verma, G.S. and Tomer, O.S. 1984. Effect of frequency of feeding on growth rates and health of Murrah buffalo calves. Indian J. Anim. Sci., 54:486-488.,

Yadav, B.S. 1982. Studies on physico-chemical properties of muscle proteins and use of tenderizing enzymes in buffaloes. Ph.D. Thesis Rohilkhand University, Bareilly.

Zeidan, M. Sedik, M.F. and Roudidy, S.A. 1976. Some studies on carcass yield of slaughtered buffaloes in Cairo abattoir. Assiut Vet. Med. J., 3:87-93 (fide Anim. Breed., Abstr., 47:2181).

Zicarelil, L., Piccolo, V., Imparato, R. and Richetti, F. 1975. Fattening and carcass characteristics of entire and castrated bufflaoes aged 30 and 42 months. Acta, Med. Vet., 21: 41-63.

Ziegler, P.T., 1964. The meat we eat. Interstate Printers and Pub., Inc., Illionois.

□□□

6

Valuable By-products of Buffalo Production and Their Utilization

Introduction

In the Bhartiya animal (Buffalo) production system all kinds of buffalo products, byproducts and waste material are utilized in different ways and for various purposes. However, economic contributions of the byproduct and waste materials are rarely accounted in the income form buffaloes by most of the small holder farmers. Accounting of the monetary value of byproducts from buffaloes, buffalo milk processing and slaughtered animals is substantial. In the present situation fo increasing cost of buffalo producs, the monetary contributions of byproducts and wste products available from the bufflaoes can not be ignored.

Kinds of Byproducts and Wastes of Buffalo Production

The byproducts and wastes of buffalo production and producs producing industries can be placed in the following foru categories.

1. **Bufflao farm byproducts:** Different kinds of byproducts and wastes of economic value are good sources of nutrients and water for the agriculture crops. Threse byproducts can be listed as follows:

   a) Buffalo dung

   b) Bufflao urine and washings: The buffalo urine mixed with the animal shed and farm washing are drained in a collection tank for the irrigation of the crops. This provision reduces environmental pollution and provides irrigation water containing some nitrogenous compounds and minerals. During dry season these farm wastes are directly driained into the fields requiring preparation for sowing.

   c) Soiled bedding

   d) Manger residue

   e) Washings

   f) Wallowing pond water

   g) Tall switch clippings

   h) Lacenta and lochea

   i) Aborted foetus

   j) Grooming dirt

2. **Dairy (milk products) byproducts:** The kinds and quantity of milk processing byproducts depend ont eh milk handling capacity and kinds of dairy products produced in the plants.

   a) Spoiled milk

   b) Spoiled and soiled milk powder

   c) Dairy utensils and equipment washing.

3. **Slaughterhouse byproducts:** Large number of buffaloes are slaughtered for meat production in unorganized and modern slaughterhouse.

a) Byproducts of unorganized and small slaughterhouses-methods of disposal.

b) Byproducts of organized abattoirs. These including following items of industrial and other uses:

i) Clean whole blood

ii) Soiled whole blood

iii) Hide

iv) Horns and hooves

v) Empty alimentary canal

vi) Lungs with wind pipe

vii) Empty gut

viii) Gut contents and urine

ix) Glands

x) Urinary bladder

xi) Channel fat

xii) Heavy bones excluded from the carcass

4. **Slaughterhouse byproducts used for biochemical and pharmaceutical extraction:** Buffalo blood, glands and some other byproducts are collected fresh, cleaned, preserved and transferred to industries for the extraction of valuable biochemicals, Pharmaceuticals and industrial products. These organs are normally collected from large slauthterhouses with adequate facilities for the collection and preservation in the premises of abattoir for transfer to industries (Table 6.1).

Table 6.1. Various byproducts and their products

Buffalo byproducts	Biochemicals, pharmaceuticals etc.
Adrenal gland	Adrenaline
Blood	Plasma, serum, albumin etc.
Fibrin	Peptone, fibrin foam, fibrin powder, bioplant etc.
Pancreases	Insulin, pancreatin, trypsinand chymotripsin
Lung and entreric mucosa	Hepatin
Liver	Liver extract (vitamins complex etc.)
Thyroid	Thyroxine
Testes	Hyaluronidase
Gall bladder	Bile, bile salts
Hair	Cardiolipins, cytochrome C
Spinal cord, brain	Cholesterol, lecithin
Bone	Gelatin, bone morphogenetic protein (BMP)
Hooves	Neats foot oil
Pituitary gland	
Anterior lobe	Follicular stimulationg hormone (FSH), leutimizing hormone (LH), ACTH, prolactin
Posterior tobe	Oxytocin, vasopressin
Ovary	Ovarian hormones

1. Buffalo farm byproducts

a) **Buffalo dung and its uses:** Buffalo dung is a daily product at the farm it has species specific strong odour which varies slightly with the quality and quantity of feds and fodders. Dung disposal is a routine practice for the maintenance of hygienic conditions. Heaps of dung provide favourable conditions for the breeding of flies, mosquitoes and beetles. The quantity of dung voided daily by buffaloes is influenced by the body size of animal, physiological state, activity, nature of the diet and level of feeding. About 10 gallon daily dung production has been reported by McGregor (141) in water buffaloes. The average faeces out put of Philippine buffaloes is about 18.8 kg daily or 6.86 tonnes annual, which contained about 43.86 per cent moisture (Vilegas, 1969). The average value for their samp buffaloes is about 18.5 kg per animal daily (Chaid *et al.*, 1983). Average daily fresh faeces production is about 26.11 (20.78-31.52) kg in Murrah buffaloes and 21.55 (20.29-22.81) kg in Vietnamese swamp buffaloes in the standard management at the farm (Pathak *et al.*, 1985). Daily faecal voided is about 0.79, 0.83 and 1.03 per cent of body weight in adult buffalo bulls, dry buffaloes and lactating buffaloes of Murrah breed. The value for adult male and female Vietnamese swamp buffaloes were 1.01 and 1.05 per cent of body weight, respectively. Annual fresh faeces production varied from 7.41 to 11.50 tonnes equivalent to 1.45 to 2.09 tonnes dry matter.

Chemical compositon of buffalo dung: The influence of the chemical composition and digestibility of feeds and fodders on the chemical composition of faeces is well known. The information considered here requresents the composition of composite manure in different conditions (Majumdar and Jung, 1963; Villegas, 1969). The content of nitrogen, phosphorus, calcium and potassium in fresh and dry faeces shows considerable nutritional value of faeces (Table 6.2) which has potential not only as manure but also as feed for livestock after suitable processing. The faeces fo Philippine buffaloes 26.14 per cent dry matter and 5.44 per cent ash. In dry faeces mean content of nitrogen, phosphorus, potash and calcium is about 0.28, 0.57, 0.11 and 0.21 per cent, respectively.

Table 6.2. Chemical composition of buffalo faeces

Faeces	Percentage of nutrients					
	Organic matter	Total ash	Nitrogen	Calcium	Phos-phorus	Potassium
Fresh basis	16-17	3-4	0.28	0.13	0.07	0.11
Dry basis	80.85	15.20	1.39	0.66	0.36	0.54

Uses of buffalo dung: Buffalo dung is one of the important sources of fuel for the domestic cooking after sun drying and manure after composting in many tropical countries. Plastering of kuccha walls and floor with a mixture of dung and clay is quite popular. The recent uses are fermentation of water diluted dung in the gobar gas (biogas) plant for the producton of fule gas, methane. The fresh dung of buffloes fed rations containing higher ratio of concentrates can be ensiled with roughates for the feeding of boine during the scarcity period for substance (Jakhnmola *et al.*, 1984). Dung cales known as upla or kanda is prepared by mixing with chaffed dry fodder wastes, free leaves, rice hulls, chaffed baggase and sugarcane trashes etc through sun drying. Dung cakes are sold for fuel int e suburban and commonly used for cooking in the rural areas. Compositon is done mistly in wet season, which drying becomes difficult. Educated and large farm families prefer composting for manure. Buffalo dung collected with soiled fodder waste and urine soaked mud is dumped in compost pits for 3-4 montsh period, where it undergoes anaerobic and aerobic microbial changes during the storage period. Organic manure not only provides nutrients to crops but also increase the moisture retention capacity of sandy soil.

Development of biogas plant has helped in reducing the pollution problems and retention of both fuel and manorial values Liquid slurry available fromt eh biogas plant 1. A richer sources of microbial protein and inorganic matter resulting from the decomposiotn of larger proportion of organic constituents for the production of methane and carbon dioxide. In addition to the manorial use, the fresh slurry of biogas plant can also be fed to supply about 20-30 per cent protein requirement for maintenance on the feeding of straw based rations (Pathak *et al.,* 1982). In recent years buffalo dung of farm animals has been made into satisfacotyr silage (wastelage) combination with chaffed straw, green fodder and a small quantity of molasses (Jakhmola *et al.,* 1984; Rameshwar Singh *et al.,* 1985). Ensiling process smay be used to make up the deficit supply of fibrous roghatges during scarcity produced by draught, flood and other fodder destroying natural calamities.

b) **Bufflao urine and washing:** Buffalo urine is a good source of non-proteinous nitrogen and it has considerable menorial value. Each litre of buffalo urine contains 9.6 -14.4 g nitrogen and 3.3 - 3.8 g potassium (Majumdar and Jung, 1963). Some portion of urine is collected with dung and solied fodder waster and substantial amount of urinary nitrogen is lost due to quick hydrolysis in the form of ammonia. Urine can also be used for the nitrogen enrichment of poor quality fodders through ensiling. On ensiling of urine soaked straw ammonia is liberated through hydrolysis by the action of natural ureas enzyme at 30-40 per cent moisture level and bind with the lignocelluloses. The alkaline thus produced contains significantly higher content of available dietary nitrogen for the ruminants and can be used for the treatment of crop residues, straws and stovers, during the scarcity period.

The buffalo urine mixed with the animal shed and farm washing are drained in a collection tank for the irrigation of the crops. This provision reduces environmental pollution and provides irrigation water containing some nitrogenous compounds and minerasl. During dry season these farm wasters are directly drained into the fields requiring preparations for soing and also in the standing crops for irriatoin. In the rainy season these wastes can be utilized for the culture of duck weeks (Azotlla and Lemna) and other aquatic platns suitable for the feeding of herbivorous and oteh ranimals. Fresh and dehydrated duck weeds are used in the diets of pigs, poultry and humans for the parital supply of crude protein and entire supply of carotenes. Some nutritious algae like chlorella and spimlina can be also grown for the dietary supplements. These algae have been incorporated in the breeds for increasing acceptability of human consumers.

c) **Use of soiled bedding and manager residue:** Bedding material used for the buffaloes are variable and depend on the local availability without any price. These include damaged straw, dry grasses, dry fallen tree leaves, dry pine needles, saw dust, wood shavings or ash. These soiled with urine and dung are collected daily alongwith coarse manger residue and dumped in the compost pits. In dry season herbal bedding s are reused for 3-4 times after sun drying and then dumped in compost pits for manure making. Oiled beddings and human manger residues produce satisfactory manure. These are also used for making dung cakes mixing with dung during the dry season.

d) **Use of wallowing pond water:** Wallowing ponds are generally drained out at weekly interval during the hot season and fortnightly interval during the cold season. The wallowing pond contaminated with urine and small amount of dung is drained out and used for the irrigation of agricultural crops. In case of community kuccha ponds (johads) used in the villages drainage is difficult. The water in such ponds is periodically diluted by adding more water fro the canals or water in such ponds is periodically diluted by adding more water from the canals or tube wells. Most of the cleaning and decontaminaton are done by the frogs and aquatic herbages.

e) **Use of plancenta, lochea and aborted foetus:** These waster products are available only during the calving season. Tehse are disposed of deep in the dung heap fo composti pit for decaying to produce manure. In some rare cases flesh of foetii aborted in advance stage during the last trimester is consumed by the humans (however, consumers do not like to be referred). Lochea and muconium (first faeces) of calves are also used in some tribal communities for the therapeutic purpose for the human and the animals.

f) **Use of tail switch clipping:** The switch of tail is made of long and coarse hairs. The switch hair is normally clipped at about 6 montsh's interval. The long and coarse hairs are used for the preparation of ropes, mats, muzzles for the animal and other useful articles like bags etc. coarse brushes of different shape and size wre quite common before the invention of synthetic fibres.

2. Dairy byproducts and wastes

The dairy byproducts and wastes not fit for human consumption are used in the foods of domestic animals.

a) **Use of spoiled milk:** Spoiled milk like sour and/or spontaneously coagulated milk is either directly fed to domestic animals after heat treatment or used for the manufacture of compounded foods for the animals.

b) **Use of spoiled/damaged milk powder:** In the manufacture of dried milk (milk powder) some amount of milk powder is soiled due to tfalling on the ground during drying and handling. The another waste is the partially charred or over heated milk powder. Both materials are used for the manufacture of compounded foods for the pet dogs and cats and also for milk replacers for the young ruminants of rumen developing stages below 8-10 weeks of age.

c) **Use of washings of the dairy or milk processing:** Washing of milk processing plants containing organic substances of milk origin which provide nuytrients for the growth of microorganisms. The washing contain different kinds of detergents and their direct drainage in the fields of standing crops may be harmful. Such washings should be made meutral or a little acidic before drainage in the fields. Diary platn washings should not be drained int eh fish ponds and natural bodies harbouring fishes, amphibian, reptiles and arthropods etc. of economic value and environmental significance.

3. Slaughterhouse byproducts

Slaughterhouse byproducts are available in small amount from the unorganized slaughters and large amount from the organized big abattoirs. In addition to these two extremes, there are semi-organized abattoris of various capacity handling 50-100 buffaloes on the 5 ir 6 working days in most parts of the country. Sacrifice of 1 or 2 buffaloes on the day of weekly market for local consumption is common in the remote village. Normally animals are slaughtered in open at a distant place from the human habitation and generally beneath a big tree. The branches of tree are frequently used as slings of hanging, flaying and dressing of the carcass. At such places there is no arrangement for the hygienic collection of byproducts for industrial uses. Almost all edible tissues of buffaloes are sold for human consumption.

Soiled blood and rejected and soiled trimmings are eaten by the stray dogs and carnivorus birds that assemble of removal of dressed carcass, head, knuckles and hide. The stray dogs and birds rush to the discarded tissues at a very fast rate. The gut and lungs with wind pipe are normally sold at the slaughter place. These are mostly purchased by the economically weaker families and used as minced meat. The entire gut is opened and thoroghyly cleaned with water. The epithelial layer of the four chambered stomach is peeled off and thrown to be eaten by stray carnivores.

In the medium and large size partially equipped and well equipped abattoris, all products and byproducts are syustematically and as far as possible hygienically collected in different lots. The valuable byproducts listed in Table 6.3. are handed over to concerned pharmaccutical industries.

Table 6.3. Buffalo slaughter byproducts from large abattoirs and their distribution to different industries.

Sl.	Byproducts	User industries
1.	Blood	Biochemical and pharmaceutical and neutraceutical industries.
2.	Glands	-do-
3.	Bones, ligaments and tendons	-do-
4.	Residues of above (1-3)	Animal feed manufacturing industries
5.	Gut	Total gastro-intestinal tract is cleaned and processed for casings manufacture for sausages.
6.	Lungs with wind pipe	Feed industry
7.	Hide	Tanneries
8.	Horns	Cottage industry
9.	Hooves	Neats oil manufacture of high quality
10.	Switch of the tail	Cottage industry
11.	Gut conent and soiled waste	Composting for manure

Use of the tissue residues of buffalo byproducts disposed of by the pharamaceutical industry: The residues of glands discarded after the extraction of hormones and enzymes and other tissues (blood, tendons, ligaments and bones etc.) are further used for the manufacture of animal feed supplements. The extracted glands residue meal is a rich source of good quality proteion. Blood residue is rich in protein and minerals and bones are the rich sources of calcium, phosphorus and magnesium.

Biochemicals, Pharmaceuticals and Neutraceuticals Products of Blood

Blood constitutes about 3 per cent of the body weight of buffaloes yielding 10-15 kg blood from the slaughtered adult buffaloes of different size.

Collection and preservation of blood for biochemical/ pharmaceutical industries

Blood for different uses are collected by the following methods at the time of slaughter.

1. **Blood collection for biochemical and pharmaceutical preparations:** Blood is collected with the use of trocar and canuls or an inoculation needle of 10 gauze in a clean and dry close container under strict hygienic conditions and sealed immediately. For the separation of plasma, an anticoagulant like sodium citrate and EDTA should be added.
2. **For the manufacture of animal feed supplements:** Blood is collected by cutting jugular vessels in clean containers and treated with calcium carbonate.
3. **For preparation of manure:** Split soiled blood is collected with other tissues in drugs and preserved with 2 per cent formalin and 2 per cent Lysol.

Various useful products of buffalo blood are presented in (Table 6.4).

Table 6.4. Products of buffalo blood

Sl.	Product	Source	Yield	Uses	Method (s)
1.	Histidine	Blood cells	1.4 %	Hoemopotesis, allergic and gastrocentreric disorders	Greenstein and Wintz, 1961)
2.	Leucine	Red blood cells	5%	Biological research, essential amino acids	-do-
3.	Lysine	-do-	1.2%	-do-	-do-
4.	Phenylal-anine	-do-	2%	-do-	-do-
5.	Haemin	Blood	0.35%	Biochemcal preparatioins	Drake and Horning, 1965
6.	Prothro-mbin	Plasma	80mg/ litre	Clinical haematology	Ansinsen, 1959, Tishkoff *et al.*,., 1978; Terlmann, 1977
7.	Thrombin	Prothro-mbin	-	Control of capillary bleeding and surgical bleeding	
8.	Fironogen	Plasma	-	Clinical haematology and therapeutics	Ingram, 1960

Fibrin and fibrin products: Foam and powder of fibrin are produced foam bovine plasma including buffalo plasma. Fibrin foam is soft and can be cut easily for dispensing in desired shape and size. It is used in surgery for arresting bleeding, Fibrin powder I also used for arresting bleeding in cases of delayed clotting.

Peptone: It is produced from different tissues like meat, alimentary canal, respiratory tract and blood protein etc. Peptone extracted from animal protein is a specialized media material for bacterial culture. It is also used for the production of bacterial toxins. Yield of peptone from meat is about 60 g per kg (Pant and Sabri, 1969).

Glandular Byproducts of Biochemcial and Therapeutic Use

Important and valuable biochemcials for research and pharmaceutical uses are extracted from different glands specially the endocrine glands. Only healthy glands are collected and processed by the industries. Following cardinal principles are followed for the collection of glands at the time of slaughter.

i) Glands are always collected fromt eh healghy animals with in 10-20 minutes of slaughter.

ii) The glands are cleaned off from connective tissues, adipose tissue and blood vessels and than cleaned immediately and frozen in solid carbon dioxide or freezing mixture.

iii) The clean and frozen glands are packed in the thermocol boxes, labeled properly and then transported to respective industries under chilled form.

Some of the commercial products manufactured from the glands and tissues are presented as follows:

Insulin: It is extracted fromt eh pancreas. Only b cells of pancreas contain insulin. Insulin is extracted from the pancreas of different species (Table 6.5), but contribution of buffaloes is greater due to the large size of pancreas.

Table 6.5. Insulin harvested from the pancreas of different species

Species	Yield/kg spleen	References
Buffalo	326 mg	Mantra *et al.*, 1980
Goat	154 mg	Yadav and Zahib Ali, 1976
Sheep	140 mg	-do-
Sheep and cattle	32.5 g	Basaba *et al.*, 1964

Heparin: Lungs, liver and mucosal tissues of alimentary tract contain high amount of heparin. It is mostly extracted from bovine lungs and intestinal mucosa of pigs. Heparin is anticoagulant and used for the prevention of blood clotting during transfusion and post operative thrombi formation.

Liver extract: In Bharat liver extract was produced by Bengal Chemicals and Pharmaceuticals, Calcutta in 1930. Adequate healthy livers are available from the organized abattoirs for the commercial manufacture of liver extract.It is used for the treatment of anemia which contains more than 0.1 mg vitamin B12 per ml.

Bile salts: Bile stored in gatt gladder is collected alongwith intact gall bladder. It is glossy greenish viscous fluid of 1.020 to 1.025 specifric gravity and slightly alkaline nature. About 500 ml. bile can be collected from 3-4 adult buffaloes or 25-30 adult goats or sheep. It is used for therapeutic purpose and biochemical research. Cholic acid of bile is used as starting material for manufacture of cortisone.

Thyroxine: Thyroid is a prominent endocrine glandwhich secrets thyroxine hormone. The desiccated gthyroid gland contsin 0.17 to 0.23% iodine. Thyroxine yield from desiceated thyroid glands is about 0.125 per cent.

Hormones of pituitary (thypophysis) gland: It is small bean shaped gland situated ina bony cavity at the base of the brain. Buffalo's pituitary gland weighs about 1.0 to 1.5 g in adult buffaloes. This has distincet antirior andposterior lobes that produce very important and essential hormones for the normal physiological functiosn of the body. The hormones of two lobes are presented as follows:

Anterior pituitary lobes: (a) Gwoth hormone (Betes *et al.*, 1940) and (b) TH and ACTH (Lietal. 1942; Sayer *et al.*, 1943).

Posterior pituitary lobe: (a) Oxytocin and (b) Vasopressin (Frankland *et al.*, 1966).

Adrenalin: It is found in adrenal gland but not extracted because synthetic adrenaline is available in the market.The adrenal glands are two pear shaped bodies each placed onteh upper border of the kidney. Adrenalin is synthesized in the medullary tissue of the gland. The concentration of adrenalin in different animals is presented in Table 6.6.

Table 6.6. Adrenalin content in glands

Species	Weight of adrenal gland (g)	Adrenal content	No. of animals for 1 kg gland
Buffalo male	11-12.5	1.83	60-70
Buffalo female	12-14	1.81	60-70
Ox	10-11	1.77	60-70
Cow	9.13	2.00	60-70
Ram	1.1-1.5	1.62	350-400
Sheep	1-1.4	1.54	350-400

Pepsin: It is a proteolyitic enzyme present in the stomach mucosa. About 200 gm abomasal mucosa lining is collected from an adult buffalo. This 7-8 g crystalline pepsin. It has therapeutic uses and also used for the tenderization of hard meat of old animals.

Cytocrome C: It is extracted from the heart tissue and used in biochemical research (Hagihara *et al.,* 1958). About 200 mg of crystalline cytochrome (C is extracted from 2 kg cardiac muscles.

Hyaluronidase: This enzyme is extracted from the testicles. It has therapeutic and biochemical uses.

Cholesterol: IT is extracted from the brain and nervous tissues (Zahid Ali, 1980). It is used in cosmetics and also for the synthesis of testosterone.

Cerebroside: It is extracted from the spinal cord of animals (Brwon and Redin, 1950).

Follicle stimulation hormone (FSH) and leutinizing hormone (LH) are present in ovaries.

Miscellaneous Products

Gelatin: Bones are the sources of gelatin which is a bone morphogenetic protein (BMP), gelatin extract method from buffalo bone has been standardized by Prasad and Kowale (1986). Defattened bones of buffaloes yield 7-8% gelatin.

Glue: It is extracted form the long bones.

Bone: residue meal: Bone residue left after extaction of gelatin or glue is used for the manufacture of sterilized bone meal for animal feed supplement or converted into manure.

Neats foot oil: It is extracted from the hooves. It is used in pharmaceutical preparatoins.About 6-7 per cent neats foot oil is extracted from the buffalo hooves (kulkarni *et al.,* 1984).

Utilization of alimentary tract: Alimentary canal from small slaughter houses is purchased by the manufacturers of food for domestic dogs, cat and zoo animals. Small intestine is also used for the manufacture of casings.

Fallen (Dead) Buffaloes Utilization

Useful disposal of dead buffaloes depends on the following conditions:

1. No. of fallen bufflaoes
2. Size of the fallen buffaloes
3. Condition of the carcass
4. Availability of the carcass utilization unit
5. Distance of carcass utilization unit and facilities for the loading, transport and unloading of carcass.

There is lack of adequate facilities for the useful disposal of 1 or 2 dead buffaloe available at weekly, fortnightly or monthly interval. Such carcasses are normally disposed of in an unhygienic manner as follows:

1. Dead buffalo is carred on sling away from the human habitations, schools, hospitals and other public places
2. Hide is removed and taken away for processing to make crude leather locally or transported to nearest tannery.
3. Most of the carcass left uncared after flying. The flesh and all soft tissues are eaten by the stray dogs, vulture, crows and other animals.
4. Bones are collected periodically and than processed for the manufacture of bone meal and bone ash. These are used as manure and stylized products are also used as mineral supplement in the diets of farm animals like poultry and pigs.
5. Heaps of gut contents are used for preparing dung cakes, manure and dried dung for fuel.

Utilization by carcass utilization industries

Some small scale cottage industries and large scale industries utilize buffalo carcass alongwith the carcass of other species for the following purposes:

1. Hide is sold to tanneries.
2. Flesh and offals including empty gut are used for the manufacture of meat meal.
3. Fascia, channel fat and other adipose tissues are used for the extraction of technical fat for soap and lubrication manufacturing industries.
4. Hooves are used for near oil extraction.
5. Horns are used in cottage industry for the manufacture of toys and utility items like comb, hair pins and button etc.
6. Bones are used for the manufacture of sterilized bone meal to be used as mineral supplements in the diets of farm animals and birds.
7. Processing wastes including gut fill are composted for manure.

References

1. Pathak, N.N. and Kamra, D.N. 1989. Agro-industrial by products, Chapter 3, pages 31-53. Processing of fibrous feeds, chapter 4, Pages 57-70. Text Book of Livestock feeding in Tropics. Casmo Publication, New Delhi.
2. Pathak, N.N. 1989. Nutritional enrichment of fibrous crop residues for livestock feeding. Centrial year of the Indian Veterinary Research Institute and Golden Jubilee year of Animal Nutrition Division, Izatnagar.

❏❏❏

7

Employment Around Buffaloes

Introduction

Domestic river buffaloes are the major dairy animals of the Indian sub-continent.Larger population of Bharat and Pakistan prefer buffalo milk as main beverage for the children and young. Among the varicty fo milk products-dahi (curd), ghee and paneer are most popular in rural as well as urban areas. Anotehr important nutritious food is the buffen (Buffalo meat). The byproducts are dung, hide, horns, hooves, glands, gut and long coarse hair sof tail switch. All the products and byproducts of the buffaloes generate chain of employment in the following four areas:

1. Rearing of buffaloes
2. Milk products, processing and marketing
3. Meat products, processing and marketing
4. Processing and marketing of byproducts

1. Buffalo Rearing

This includes calf rearing, replacement stock rearing, fattening, breeding buffaloes rearing and spent buffaloes rearing. The employment avenues are grazing, wallowing management, feeding on the stall, grooming, maintenance of housing, milking, milk utilization, dung collection and processing, fattening of spared male calves and marketing of each product. Although in the prevalent system of buffalo rearing estimationof working hours and the number of animal managed byu a personof more persons. However, an assessment has been made onteh basis of meager information available. The standards of government buffalo farm are not applicable to families rearing only few buffaloes and their followers for livelihood.

Kinds of employment in buffalo rearing

The part time engagement of family members is normally not accounted in the inputs on buffalo rearing. The works carried by the owners may include.

a) Collection of dung and disposal at a fixed place. This is done normally three times daily in case of stall fed animals and twice daily in the grazing animals.

b) Feeding of buffaloes is also done twice daily in early morning and later afternoon in stall fed and only once in morning in grazing animals. The duration of adequate grazing to satiety is generally 4 to 6 months of wet rainy season in most parts of the country.

c) Preparation of concentrates includes grinding of grains, mixing of the feed ingredients and soaking in water for 6-8 hours. Cooking of concentrate mixture is also practiced in many parts of Bharat, Nepal and Pakistan.

d) Milking of the lactating buffaloes twice daily. Rarely thrice daily in few animals yielding 20 kg or more milk daily.

e) Grooming and washing of buffaloes is normally not required for the adult allowed wallowing.

f) Sale of milk at the milk collectoni cintres of cooperative societies, some other dairies, halwai or door delivery.

g) Processing of milk for the preparation of curd, makhan, ghee khoa or mawa, chhena and paneer etc.

h) Feeding and cleaning of young calves retained at door of preventing suckling during grazing. The calves are allowed limited suckling for letdown of milk at the morning after noon milking.

i) Occasional works include breeding of females in heat, care of sick animal (s), seasonal vaccination, periodic dewarming and sale of surplus animals at door or in the bazaar and fairs for the animals. These works are also carried by the hired workers.

Casual jobs of regular continuity

a) A person managed 15-20 adult buffloes on growing and browsing in a group of 3 to 5 persons managing a herd 50 to 100 buffaloes for 8-10 hours on grazing lands and wallowing ponds or other available water sources like river, streams, lakes and canals etc.

b) A milker handles 8-10 buffaloes for moning and evening milking

c) Cleaning of buffalo house, mangers and yard: A casual worker attends 1 to 10 holds depending on the number of animals. The job includes collecton and disposal of dung, rejected feed residue and bedding (if used) at a fixed place and cleaning the premises.

2. Milk Marketing

Consumption of fluid buffalo milk is quite common in the Indian sub-continetn and almost entire urban population purchase fluid milk either formthe producers' door at the time of milking or from other sources. The fluid milk in rural areas is either collected by vendors (milk man or dudhia) from door to door for sale or processed by the producers for the sale of products.

Milk marketing by vendors/ dudhias: This is a diverse class of people handling 50 to 100 kg fluid milk in metallic cans for a distance of less than 10 km to more than several hundread kilometer like Rajasthan to Kolkata. The containers used are metallic cans, milk tanker and rail tankers. The tankers carrying milk for long distance are refrigerated for preventing coagulation of fluid milk.

Milk processing and marketing by the milk processing dairies: The large dairy plants handle thousand litre of milk for marketing as fluid milk in different quantity of polypacks and other containers. The milk collected at the dairies is standardized as whole milk, toned milk,double tones milk and skim milk. Long age glass bottles with red, blue and yellow aluminum caps were used for denoting cow milk, buffalo milk and skim milk, respectively. Now, polypacks with inscription in different colours denote the milk content.

3. Milk Products Manufacture and Marketing

This ranges from individual household to cottage industries, traditional halwais and large milk products manufacturing dairies and factories. The products are cream, butter, curd, srikhand, ghee, paneer, cheese, khoa and several arieties of sweets.

Kinds of employment in milk and milk products manufacture and marketing

Different kinds of part time and full time employment are avaialbe in the milk processing, milk product manufacture and marketing. These include :

a) Fluid milk collection from small hoders.

b) Transportation of milk to collection centres, chilling plants, milk processing dairies, halwais and other consumers.

c) Skilled manpower for the manufacture of milk products.

d) Packaging of milk and milk products in different kinds of containers of wholesale and retain shops.

e) Transporation of milk and milk products to wholesale and retail shops in local market and other cities and town.

4. Other jobs Producing Industries Associated with Buffalo Production and Products Manufacture and Marketing

a) Farmers engaged in cultivation and sale of green fodder, dry fodder, cereal grains, pulses and oilseeds etc.

b) Food grain and oil seeds milling plants providing bran, rice polish,pulses milling byproducts like hulls, husk and chunni and oilseeds milling plants producing oil seed cakes for livestock feeding.

c) Compounded feed manufacturing industries producing concentrates mixtures for different classes of dairy and other farm animals directly or indirectly associated with the dairy industries.

d) Milk containers manufacturing units ranging fromlocal earthern pots milking artisan to large milk carriers loaded onteh trucks and rails.

e) Manufacture of milk processing andproducts making utensils to large size machines for the manufacture of ghee, cheese, dried milk powder and casein etc.

f) Manufacture of milk and milk products packaging materials and their lebeling.

g) Cooling machines of different size from freeze to deep freeze and others used for transporation, storage, retail shops and also required for small units of mobile vendors.

h) Vehicles for transporation of animals, feed and fodder, milk and milk products etc. These range from head load to sling, bicycle, rickshwaw, tempo, mini truck, truck, tankers and rail wagons. In very remote areas pack animals, animal driven carts, boats and steamers are also used.

f) Processing of dung for the preparation of dung cakes of different shape and size for fuel and composting of dung with other organic wastes for manure preparation.

j) Disposal and recycling of wastes and scraps etc.

All these steps in mil production, processing and marketing provide different kinds of skilled and unskilled demployment for illiterate persons to highly qualified skilled persons without any reserveation to cost, creed and gender. The jobs are generated from remote areas to compolitan cities. Even the yak nanaging Brokpa tribe of cold zone prepare yak milk products like ghee, butter and churpee for sale in markets of foot hills. Bangaries rear buffaloes in deep forest and Vangwzzars on the high Himalayan Bugyals (pastures of summer season)_prepare ghee and butter for sale in the plains and other market.

5. Meat production and Marketing

The fattened surplus males, sterile heifers, spent females, inactive buffalo bulls and retired working buffloes are slaughtered for meat, blood, gands, hide, horns, hooves and switch of the tail.

Meat production includes slughter, bleeding, dressing and partitioning of carcass in whole sale cuts. The amin products for specialized marketing are :

a) Carcass without glands or wish kidneys for the meat markets.

b) Blood and glands for the pharmaceutical and other industries.

c) Hides for leather manufacturing industry (Tannery) and ultimately for leather goods making industry

d) Horns and hair sof tail switch for cottage industry

e) Sortings, hooves and gut switch for cottage industry

Out of these five groups, first three generate chain of works that provide different kinds of skilled and unskilled jobs. These materials are processed in big as well as cottage industries. The market range for these products is quite large and extends in other coutnreis also.

Employment in byproducts utilization: Many valuable byproducts provide employment (part time and full time) large number of skilled and unskilled manpower or rural and urban areas.

Area of employment: By products and wastes available from the buffaloes provide employment for the following workds

a) Collection of dung and yard refuse.

b) Dumping of dung and yard refuse in the manure pints for composting.

c) Removal, transportation and dispersal of manure in the fields before plouging and sowing.

d) Preparatoin and marketing of buffalo dung alone or dung mixed with other byproducts and wastes like saw dust, fallen dry tree leaves and fine residues of coal etc.

e) Flaying of skin of dean buffaloes.

f) Manufacture of meat meal, meat-cum-bone meal, bone meal and bnoe ash etc. for supplemental feeding of pigs and poulutry, Bone meal and bone ash are mineral supplements for the farm animal and also used as manures.

g) Horne and hooves are used for the extraction of good quality oil for lubrication of machines. The horns are used for the manufacture of fancy and daily use articles like comb, stuck, toys, hair pins, button etc. Sortings are composted for manure. Collection, sorting and disposal of hide, horns, hooves, blood and gut contents from the slaughtered buffaloes.

h) Processign of hide for leather making.

i) Manufacture of varieties of leather goods for domestic and export markets.

j) Colelction, cleaning and marketing of blood, serum and glands for the manufacture of pharmaceuticals, neutraceutical and cosmetics etc.

6. Export of Buffalo Products

Some of the important buffalo products exposed insubstantial quantity are :

a) Whole carcass for table meat

b) Different kinds of buffalo meat products

c) Buffalo leather and leather goods

d) Fancy and decoration articles made of buffalo horns.

e) Pharamaceuticals manufacture from the glands.

Export of buffalo products is an important source of foreign exchange earning in hard currency.

7. Future of buffaloes and Employment around Buffaloes

With the graph of human population growth in most of the buffalo rearing coutnreis, the requirement of good quality protein will continue to increase. Buffalo meat (buffen) is widely acceptable and large number of consumer are also present in the Bharat. The demand of buffen and buff-veal will further increase on the display of essential amino acids composition of buffalo flesh and cholesterol content in the edible carcass compared with the flesh of other meat producing animals. The quantity of most of the essential amino acids in buffalo meat is much higher in comparison to meat of many other mammalaian species. Cholesterol content in buffen and bull-veal is quite low in comparison to other table meats.

Therefore, future of buffalo product is quite bright and it will continue to provide variety of employment. The part time and whole time jobs around the buffalo production provide employment from children to senior persons depending on their health and physical conditions. The jobs are diversified and start from procurement and rearing of the buffaloes to processing and marketing of the products.

❑❑❑

Subject Index

❑❑❑